STRESS
and the
FAMILY

VOLUME I:
Coping With
Normative Transitions

Edited by

Hamilton I. McCubbin &
Charles R. Figley

BRUNNER/MAZEL, *Publishers* • New York

Library of Congress Cataloging in Publication Data

Main entry under title:

Stress and the family.

   Vol. 2 edited by Charles R. Figley & Hamilton I.
McCubbin.
   Includes bibliographies and indexes.
   Contents: v. 1. Coping with normative transitions
—v. 2. Coping with catastrophe.
   1. Family—Addresses, essays, lectures.
2. Stress (Psychology)—Addresses, essays, lectures.
I. McCubbin, Hamilton I. II. Figley, Charles R.,
1944-   . [DNLM: 1. Stress, Psychological.
2. Life change events. 3. Family. WM 172 S9136]

HQ734.S9735 1983   306.8'5   83-6048
ISBN 0-87630-321-1 (v. 1)
ISBN 0-87630-332-7 (v. 2)

SECOND PRINTING

Copyright © 1983 by Hamilton I. McCubbin and Charles R. Figley

Published by

BRUNNER/MAZEL, INC.
19 Union Square West
New York, N.Y. 10003

MANUFACTURED IN THE UNITED STATES OF AMERICA

Dedicated to

our family friends,
Reuben and Marion Hill,

and our families,
Marilyn, Todd, Wendy and Laurie,
and
Marilyn and Jessica

Preface to the Series

As editors of this two-volume series, we are delighted to introduce the reader to a burgeoning area of research in the social sciences: family stress and coping. The books view the family as both producing and reacting to stress and attempt to identify the sources of stress from either inside or outside the family microsystem. Further, the volumes distinguish between sudden, unpredictable, and overwhelming catastrophic stress and the more "normal," gradual, and cumulative life stressors encountered over the life span. Moreover, the series brings into focus several rich perspectives which effectively integrate the hundreds of generalizations about the functional and dysfunctional methods family members use to cope with stress.

We hope that these volumes will be a unique contribution to the collection of publications already in print or in press by providing conceptual clarity and scholarly direction. This series represents an area of inquiry which has emerged quite recently, though early elements date back over a half-century. We build upon the important contributions of Reuben Hill, Hans Selye, Richard Lazarus, Mardi Horowitz, and many others in an attempt to synthesize the relevant research into an organized set of empirical generalizations. These are designed, among other things, to stimulate new hypotheses and innovations in research and intervention in this growing area.

Moreover, we hope that this series will help move the field of family studies forward by viewing family stress as a predictable aspect of family development and change over the life span. In this preface let us briefly discuss our purpose, beliefs, objectives, organizational structure, and how this nearly three-year enterprise was conceived and produced.

PURPOSE AND BELIEFS

The purpose of the series is to organize a compendium of empirically-based observations about the ways families produce, encounter, and cope with stress. The intended readers include students and professionals interested in understanding and helping people within the family context.

From the beginning we want our values known; by doing so we alert the reader to the presence of potential bias in our efforts to relate the facts as we find them. For instance, we believe that family members often know better than anyone else what is best for them and their family—better than clinicians, professors, advice column writers and other experts, for example. We also believe that the role of "helping" families is one of helping families attain goals, helping families experience the kind of life together they wish to have, though it may be different from what we wish for our own families. Finally, we believe that consulting with families is superior to directing them, and educating families is superior to indoctrinating them.

OBJECTIVES

In an effort to explicate the nature and consequences of stress for people living within families, we intend that our volumes reach five specific objectives:

(a) to clearly define and provide a framework for viewing the family system as both a stress absorber as well as a stress producer;

(b) to explicate the key concepts and variables associated with this framework;

(c) to identify the important areas of research inquiry which converge into the family stress area of study that facilitates the development of a discrete set of axioms toward which a theory of family stress can be built;

(d) to note the effective strategies of intervention by professionals to either mitigate or ameliorate the impairments of family stress; and

(e) to clearly identify the various sources of stress, stress reactions of family members, stress-coping resources, repertoire, and behaviors.

ORGANIZATIONAL STRUCTURE

The reader should be aware by now that *Stress and the Family* is divided into two volumes. The first volume, *Coping with Normative Transitions*, focuses on the everyday stressors families experience, especially those many transitions throughout the life cycle as family relationships change and family members grow and develop. The second volume, *Coping with Catastrophe*, focuses on the extraordinary stressors which strike families suddenly and often overwhelm the family's ability to cope. In each volume, chapters are organized into roughly two groups by the locus of family stressors: either from inside the family system (e.g., birth of a child, death in the family) or from outside the family system (e.g., economic inflation, unemployment).

A large collection of noted experts in various areas have been commissioned to write chapters which utilize the family stress framework to answer 10 questions:

1) What is the family stressor which is the focus of the chapter?
2) Why should there be an interest in this stressor?
3) What are some precepts/principles which make it easier to understand and appreciate the complexities and methods of coping with this stressor?
4) What are the elements of this stressor which are upsetting and require those affected to develop methods of coping?
5) What are the typical, dysfunctional methods individuals and families employ to deal with this source of stress?
6) What are the typical, functional methods of coping?
7) What are the resources available to the family system which are so effective in coping with the stressor?
8) What are some practical prescriptions for dealing with this stressor?
9) What are the effective methods employed by professionals and clinicians to help people and their families cope?
10) How can dysfunctional stress reactions be prevented?

Chapters 1, 10, and 15 in Volume I and Chapters 1 and 11 in Volume II, in addition to the introductions to the volumes, provide important conceptual clarity in an attempt to present an overview of the chapters that follow them. Definitions and discussions of critical concepts and synthesizing models and frameworks are found within these chapters.

HISTORY AND EMERGENCE OF THIS SERIES

To date, these two volumes are the first attempts to provide a textbook for students and professionals interested in a comprehensive under- standing of stress and the family. Scholarly discussions of individual and family stress, however, have appeared in a wide range of behavioral, social, and medical publications for the past 60 years. Traditionally, these studies and clinical observations have been limited in scope, focusing on individuals exclusively or isolated circumstances of families in stress- ful situations. In addition, these previous works tend to underscore the dysfunctional and deleterious effects of stressful life events.

This two-volume series attempts to clarify the nature and processes of family adjustment to stress, with a deliberate and well-placed em- phasis on family coping and support. The emergence of this series is due, in part, to the special chemistry which results in the collaboration between colleagues from different scholarly disciplines and interests. Figley is a family psychologist with special interests in how human beings react to traumatic events within the context of the family. McCubbin is a family psychologist with special interest in the family system's reactions to stress mediated by its members' coping responses and community supports. Together we share many basic assumptions about stress and the family, yet differ in our approach to many issues within this area. The former, for example, is more concerned about the clinical intervention implications and the latter more interested in the conceptualization and measurement issues.

Our collaboration dates back to 1975 when we served as co-panelists in a research symposium on the family readjustment problems of re- turning Vietnam veterans. We were each working in the same area, but within different contexts. Dr. McCubbin was Head of the Family Studies Branch of the Center for POW Studies at the Naval Health Research Center in San Diego. There he directed a major study of the impact of father absence and initial impact of his return among the families of prisoners of war and those missing in action during the Vietnam war. At the same time, Dr. Figley was studying the emotional upheavals associated with the war by studying Vietnam combat veterans and their families in his capacity as founder and director of the Consortium on Veteran Studies at Purdue University.

In 1976 we began to speculate together and separately about the stres- sors of separation and reunion associated with war, building upon the nearly 30 years of pioneering work of Reuben Hill. Less than four years later we, along with a dozen other colleagues, formed the Task Force on Families of Catastrophe to assist the U.S. State Department in efforts to care for the families of American personnel trapped in Iran between November, 1979, and January, 1981. At that time we applied what we had learned about the families affected by wars and other traumatic events. We became convinced that a textbook was needed which could pull together the family stress research literature not only to help policy makers and interventionists working with families in crisis, but for the field in general.

The first step in that direction was the 1980 Groves Conference on Marriage and the Family with the theme, "Stress and the Family." Dr. Figley served as program chair and Dr. McCubbin delivered the keynote address. It was from this conference, held in Gatlinburg, Tennessee in May, 1980, that many of the initial ideas and organizational structure of this series emerged. For example, many of the chapters contributed to both volumes (Chapters 2-5 and 12 in Volume I and Chapters 1, 4, 5, and 10 in Volume II) were presented in some form at this four-day seminal conference. Indeed, because of its conception within the Groves Conference and the importance of this society of family scholars and practitioners to future contributions to the social sciences, all royalties from the sale of these volumes are being donated to the Groves Foundation. These and other funds will enable the Groves Conference to continue to sponsor innovative and lively symposia each year, bringing together students of the family to consider the past and present and to speculate on the future as it has for nearly 50 years.

We hope that you enjoy the series and can begin soon to apply its lessons in whatever context is of importance to you.

Hamilton I. McCubbin
Charles R. Figley

Acknowledgments

This volume would not have been possible were it not for the help of those who shared our commitment to understanding families under stress.

My co-editor, Charles Figley, has long been a colleague and friend, and a prime mover in this project. His skill as a scholar and an editor will long be appreciated by me.

We would not have been able to manage the challenge of integrating the various perspectives into a meaningful whole without the editorial work of Catherine Davidson at the University of Minnesota. Her patience, kindness, and thoroughness played a major part in smoothing out the rough edges and in giving the volume a touch of class. I would also like to thank Joan Patterson, who took the time and offered her professional skills in reviewing several manuscripts.

I am very appreciative of the assistance given to us by key administrators at the University of Minnesota. I would like to thank Dr. Richard Sauer, Director, Agricultural Experiment Station, University of Minnesota, who gave this project the support it needed to see its way to completion. I would also like to acknowledge the continued support and patience of Dean Keith McFarland, and Associate Dean Signe Betsinger of the College of Home Economics at the University of Minnesota. Their encouragement was, as always, greatly appreciated.

Because this volume was prepared in part during a sabbatical leave, I would like to thank the University of Minnesota for allowing me this respite from academic and administrative duties and for continuing commitment to scholarship. I would also like to thank Gardner Lindzey, Director of the Center for Advanced Studies in the Behavioral Science at Stanford University for providing a nurturing setting to pursue the completion of this volume while serving as a summer scholar at the Center.

I am also indebted to the faculty and staff of the Department of Family Social Science, especially to Gloria Lawrence, Jane Schwanke, Todd

McCubbin, Susan Rains-Johnson, Kay Lapour, Emma Haugan, Alida Malkus, and Dorothea Berggren for their assistance in manuscript preparation.

I am very grateful to those scholars who served as referees of the papers in this book. Their special expertise contributed greatly to the quality of scholarship. Our thanks to Professors Linda Budd, James Maddock, Jeylan Mortimer, Ronald Pitzer and Paul Rosenblatt of the University of Minnesota; Professor William Doherty, of the University of Iowa; Professor Francille Firebaugh of Michigan State University; Professor Beatrice Paolucci of Ohio State University; and Professor Candyce Russell of Kansas State University. I would especially like to thank Professor Laura Smart of Northern Illinois University for her careful reading of the entire volume and for her suggestions on style and organization, which improved the readability of the book.

Hamilton I. McCubbin
University of Minnesota

The enterprise of scholarly inquiry can be an exciting and worthwhile venture, as the reader will discover in this volume. What is less obvious are the numerous individuals who have contributed so much of their time and talent to the creation of this volume.

As noted elsewhere, my collaboration with Hamilton McCubbin spans nearly a decade. We have become trusted friends and colleagues over the years, especially during the process of co-editing the two volumes in this series. His international stature as a family stress scholar is clearly evident throughout this volume and I am deeply indebted to him for his inspirational contributions as well as his editorial expertise.

The Groves Conference on Marriage and the Family deserves special acknowledgment. This society was the first to see the importance of the concept of stress and its relevance to the family and commissioned a national conference on the topic. Many of the chapters in this volume were conceived as a result of that conference.

It would have been nearly impossible to undertake and complete this massive project without the cooperation and assistance of so many at Purdue University. Dr. Norma Compton, Dean of the School of Consumer and Family Sciences, Dr. Billy R. Baumgardt, Director of the Agricultural Experiment Station, and Dr. Robert A. Lewis, Head of the Department of Child Development and Family Studies, provided critical administrative support and encouragement. The faculty of the Department of Child Development and Family Studies and the Child and Family Research Institute were extremely important in the development and completion of the project in various capacities: contributors, reviewers, or sources of encouragement. Also I appreciate the clerical help of Roberta Thayer, Karen Hinkley, and Barbara Brecker, as well as the support with various tasks from my graduate students, Joan Jurich, Richard Kishur, and Sandra Burge. But the key person in the project who helped bring it to fruition was Vicki Hogancamp, who served at various times as conference coordinator for the conference on "Stress and the Family," editorial assistant, and co-author of one of the chapters in the series. Ms. Hogancamp's extraordinary skills and professionalism were clearly evident in her success at assisting the editors in critiquing, organizing, rewriting, editing, and typing a considerable portion of this volume.

We are also indebted to those who helped us read and review manuscripts, bringing to the task their special expertise on the various topics discussed in this book. Our thanks to Jan Allen, Arthur Blank, Veda Boyer, Bernard Bloom, Ann Wolbert Burgess, Michael Clapman, Richard Clayton, Barbara Dahl, Thomas Drabeck, Robert Fetsch, Richard Gelles, Harold Hackney, Donald Hartsough, James Huber, Anthony Jurich, Daniel Lonnquist, Phyllis Moen, Thomas Saarinen, Nancy Sederberg, Graham Spanier, M. Duncan Stanton, Dena Targ, Richard Venjohn and William Yarber. We would especially like to thank Laura Smart for her careful reading of the entire manuscript and her excellent suggestions on style and organization, which improved the readability of both volumes in the series.

I would also like to acknowledge several colleagues who were helpful to me during my sabbatical leave, enabling me to complete work on the series by providing resources of their respective institutions and the stimulation of their respective minds: Ann Wolbert Burgess, Boston University Medical School; Robert Rich, the Woodrow Wilson School of Public and International Affairs, Princeton University; and John Talbott, Payne-Whitney Clinic, Department of Psychiatry, Cornell Medical College.

Charles R. Figley
Purdue University

Contents

Contributors

Constance Ahrons, Ph.D.
Associate Professor, School of Social Work, University of Wisconsin, Madison.

Marc Baranowski, Ph.D.
Associate Professor, Department of Child Development and Family Relations, University of Maine, Orono.

Pauline Boss, Ph.D.
Associate Professor, Department of Family Social Science, University of Minnesota, St. Paul.

Cheryl Buehler, Ph.D.
Assistant Professor, Department of Child and Family Studies, University of Tennessee, Knoxville.

Raymond T. Coward, Ph.D.
Professor and Research Director, Center for Rural Studies, University of Vermont, Burlington.

Richard M. Dunham
Associate Professor, Department of Psychology, Florida State University.

Charles R. Figley, Ph.D.
Professor and Director, Child and Family Research Institute, Purdue University, West Lafayette.

Judith L. Fischer
Associate Professor Department of Home and Family Life, Texas Tech. University.

Mary Ann Noecker Guadagno, Ph.D.
Assistant Professor in the Department of Family Social Science, University of Minnesota, St. Paul.

M. Janice Hogan, Ph.D.
Associate Professor, Department of Family Social Science, University of Minnesota, St. Paul.

Robert W. Jackson
Extension Associate Professor and Program Coodinator, Extension Home Economics, Vermont Extension Service.

Jeannie Kidwell, Ph.D.
Professor, Department of Child and Family Studies, University of Tennessee, Knoxville.

Harriette P. McAdoo, Ph.D.
Professor, School of Social Work, Howard University, Washington, D.C., and Research Associate at Columbia Research Systems.

Hamilton I. McCubbin, Ph.D.
Professor and Head, Department of Family Social Science, University of Minnesota, St. Paul.

Gail F. Melson, Ph.D.
Professor, Department of Child Development and Family Studies, Purdue University, West Lafayette.

Brent C. Miller, Ph.D.
Associate Professor, Department of Family and Human Development, Utah State University, Logan.

Judith A. Myers-Walls, Ph.D.
Extension Specialist in Human Development, Purdue University, West Lafayette.

Gerhard Neubeck, Ph.D.
Professor, Department of Family Social Science, University of Minnesota, St. Paul.

Joan M. Patterson, M.S.
Doctoral Candidate and Research Associate, Department of Family Social Science, University of Minnesota, St. Paul.

Joyce Portner, Ph.D.
Associate Director, Continuing Education in Social Work, University of Minnesota, Minneapolis.

Beatrice Robinson, M.S.
Doctoral Candidate, Department of Family Social Science, University of Minnesota, St. Paul.

Denise A. Skinner, Ph.D.
Assistant Professor, Department of Human Development, University of Wisconsin, Stout.

Emily Visher, Ph.D.
Clinical Psychologist in private practice, Palo Alto, California.

John Visher, M.D.
Psychiatrist and Head of Adult Services, North County Mental Health Center of the San Mateo County Community Mental Health Division, California.

Kaye L. Zuengler, R.N., M.S.
Doctoral Candidate, Department of Family Social Science, University of Minnesota, St. Paul.

Introduction

To talk of "normal" stressors and crises, the subject of this first volume of *Stress and the Family*, sounds like a contradiction in terms. How can a stressor or a crisis be "normal"? Most of us think of stress as a result of an extreme or unusual event, like the catastrophes we discuss in Volume II—war, death, fire, unemployment, and so on. But we also know that family life is constantly changing, even if the changes—the birth of a child, a parent getting a new job—are expected, predictable, and happen to almost everyone. These changes still require ongoing adjustment and adaptation by family members and the family system, often just as much adjustment as a sudden extraordinary event. Thus normative stressors and crises refer to those changes or transitions which are expected and predictable, which most or even all families will experience over the life cycle, and which require adjustment and adaptation.

These normal stressors and crises occur because family members and the family system change over time in normal social, psychological, and physical development. Stress is part of that developmental process. Family scholars have sought to understand the nature of these stressful transitions and how families effectively and ineffectively cope with them. This volume attempts to shed light upon these stressors and the overall process of family coping.

Before discussing the various chapters in this book, we will expand on this concept of "normative transition."

NORMATIVE LIFE CYCLE TRANSITIONS

The concept of normative life transitions is a key idea behind the chapters in this book. Theorists of human development have provided insight into how families change over the life cycle. There appear to be three aspects of normative transitions in the family, each with its own separate yet interlocking set of demands: individual development, gender-specific development, and family development. The demands or tasks at each stage are major sources of stress.

Individual Development

The classic work of Erik Erikson (1950, 1976) has made us more aware of the key psychosocial "crises" each of us experiences over the life span. For Erikson, a developmental crisis is "a turning point, a crucial period of increased vulnerability and heightened potential" (Golan, 1981, p. 26). Like other theorists of development, Erikson posits that the degree to which an individual resolves a given crisis can either enhance or weaken his or her ability to resolve or master subsequent ones. Erikson sees eight crisis points in the life cycle, each with its own conflicting demands and key critical element or antidote needed to resolve the crisis. For example, the infant struggles with the crisis of "trust versus mistrust" and overcomes it through "hope." The infant develops trust in his parents; the feelings of hope allow the infant to let the mother out of sight without anxiety. The mother has become "an inner certainty as well as an outer predictability" (Erikson, 1950, p. 247). Once the child trusts the parents, he or she builds on this trust and begins to seek greater independence (autonomy vs. shame; initiative vs. guilt), and later moves to master certain skills and develop relationships with peers (industry vs. inferiority). The adolescent must deal with the developmental task of establishing a personal identity (identity vs. identity confusion) (See Table 1).

TABLE 1
Personal Psychosocial Crises

STAGE	CONFLICT	RESOLUTION
Infancy	Trust vs. mistrust	HOPE
Early Childhood	Autonomy vs. shame, doubt	WILL
Play Age	Initiative vs. guilt	PURPOSE
School Age	Industry vs. inferiority	COMPETENCE
Adolescence	Identity vs. identity confusion	FIDELITY
Young Adulthood	Intimacy vs. isolation	LOVE
Maturity	Generativity vs. self-absorption	CARE
Old Age	Integrity vs. despair, disgust	WISDOM

Adapted from Erik H. Erikson, *Adulthood* (New York: W. W. Norton & Co., 1976), p. 25.

Erikson saw adult development beginning with the commitment to another (intimacy vs. isolation), moving to a mature stage in the development of a productive work or family life (generativity vs. self-absorption), and then to the resolution of one's life in old age (integrity vs. despair). Other theorists have concentrated specifically on expanding this framework of individual adult development (Havighurst, 1953; see Table 2), some seeing variations in the patterns for men (Levinson et al., 1978) and women (Sanguilano, 1978).

Since most of us, adults and children, struggle with these life crises within families, it is important to understand that a psychosocial crisis for one family member is often stressful for other family members. The parents may be going through one kind of developmental crisis, while the children are going through another. In other words, the developmental needs of family members may overlap and complement one another, or they may conflict or compete with one another. "Cogwheeling," that is, the fitting together of the developmental cycles of individual family members, appears to be a central concept in explaining how

TABLE 2
Adult Developmental Tasks

Early Adulthood (18-35)

Select a mate.	Manage a home.
Learn to live with a marriage partner.	Get started in an occupation.
	Take on civic responsibility.
Start a family.	Find a congenial social group.
Rear children.	

Middle Age (35-60)
Achieve adult civic and social responsibility.
Establish and maintain an economic standard of living.
Assist teenage children to become responsible and happy adults.
Develop adult leisure-time activities.
Relate oneself to one's spouse as a person.
Accept and adjust to the physiological changes of middle age.
Adjust to aging parents.

Later Maturity (60 and over)
Adjust to decreasing physical strength and health.
Adjust to retirement and reduced income.
Adjust to death of spouse.
Establish an explicit affiliation with one's age group.
Meet social and civic obligations.
Establish satisfactory physical living arrangements.

From R. Havighurst, *Human Development and Education*. London, England: Longmans, Green, 1953, pp. 757-283.

individual developmental tasks mesh with one another in the family system. For example, a husband might want to spend more time in the family in his quest for generativity (Erickson's seventh stage); this may compete with his wife's struggle for self-expression that her new career provides or with his teenage children's efforts to gain identity by moving away from the family unit. The stress of family life in this situation is obvious.

Gender-Specific Developmental Tasks

Another developmental theorist, Klaus Riegel (1976), has pointed out there are differences in developmental tasks for men and women. Riegel sees development from a dialectical perspective: Changing events within the person's thoughts, actions, and emotions are seen as influencing events in the outer world of the family and community. Simultaneously, the changes in the outer world influence the events within the individual and his immediate environment (like his family). From the interaction between the inner and the outer spheres, human development occurs. Riegel draws a distinction between the timing of psychosocial and biophysical changes for males and females, which has not been fully considered by other theorists. But given the different sex-role socialization for men and women in our society, and the different social definitions of masculine and feminine behavior, it is hardly surprising that male and female development should differ in some ways.

For both sexes, Riegel suggests six distinct stages in the adult years, starting at age 20. Table 3 illustrates his framework. Stage I is a time of education, first job, marriage and first child. Very frequently the first child is the demarcation point for career-oriented couples who ordinarily wish for and attempt to develop an egalitarian relationship which implies like experiences. Yet in most instances the work patterns of women are more disrupted by the birth of a child and, indeed, throughout the childrearing years than the work life of men. The other stages and the sudden changes common to both are noted in Table 3.

These normative predictable life cycle transitions serve as the complex background for families coping with other kinds of changes, the catastrophes of life. These catastrophes are the subject of Volume II of *Stress and the Family*.

TABLE 3

Family-Adult Developmental Tasks: Men and Women

LEVEL (Years)	Males		Females		Sudden Changes
	Psychosocial	Biophysical	Psychosocial	Biophysical	
I(20-25)	college/first job	marriage	marriage	first child	
II(25-30)	first child second job other children		loss of job	other children	
III(30-35)	children in preschool move	promotion	without job		
IV(35-50)	children in school second home	promotion departure of children	second career departure of children	menopause	loss of job loss of parents loss of friends illness
V(50-65)	unemployment isolation	grandfather head of kin incapacitation	grandmother head of kin unemployment	widowhood incapacitation	retirement
VI(65 +)	deprivation	sensory-motor deficiencies			loss of partner death

From K. Riegel. Adult Life Crises: A Dialectical Interpretation of Development. In N. Datan & L. H. Ginsberg (Eds.), *Life Span Developmental Psychology: Normative Life Crises*, New York: Academic Press, 1975, pp. 123-126.

NORMATIVE FAMILY STRESS RESEARCH: AN
OVERVIEW OF VOLUME I

The contributors to this volume are either researchers or counselors
who focus on various sources or facets of family stress and coping. Most
are professors who have made important contributions in their various
areas of specialization, which are, in fact, sources of stress for the family:
divorce, pregnancy and childbirth, adolescence, sexuality, or marital
interaction, for example. Each contributor was asked to write a chapter
which fully described the significance of the family stressors they were
discussing in terms of (a) the extent or impact of a stressor on individuals
and families; (b) the characteristic patterns of coping by the family and
family members which helped or hindered adjustment or adaptation;
and (c) the implications of this information for policymakers or psycho-
therapists who wished to assist families coping with stress.

The various authors do not offer a unified perspective on stress and
coping. They write about each of the stressors from their own perspective, and these perspectives differ theoretically, methodologically, clin-
ically, and philosophically. For example, Emily and John Visher would
reject the whole notion of the nuclear family as an ideal, because they
feel it prevents stepfamilies from taking a positive view of stepfamily
life. Constance Ahrons, however, would build on the concept of the
nuclear family to generate the idea of the "binuclear family" to explain
the process of divorce in families. Some writers, such as Kidwell and
her colleagues, view coping from the viewpoint of systems theory, while
others, such as Noecker Guadagno, use a family management framework to understand coping.

This range of differences in assumptions and theories associated with
stress and the family demonstrates an important point. For all of us, but
especially for students and young professionals, this diversity of perspectives can contribute to our understanding of stress and the family,
and demonstrate how much opportunity there is for scholars and practitioners to study, add to, and apply the principles of normative family
change.

In spite of these differences in perspective, it is remarkable how much
similarity these scholars see in how families respond to different stressors. The methods of functional coping are very similar across the different transitions and demands. These coping strategies include seeking
information and understanding of the stressor event; seeking social support from relatives, friends, neighbors, others in similar situations, and

professionals; being flexible about family roles; taking an optimistic view of the situation; and improving family member communication.

The chapters in this book are divided into two parts: Part I on *Family Transitions* begins with a theoretical chapter which outlines basic concepts, followed by eight chapters which each focus on one stressor or set of stressors around family transitions. Part II on *Environmental Demands on the Family* begins with a theoretically oriented chapter, followed by four chapters focusing on different sets of normative stressors from outside the family. The final chapter attempts to synthesize the major points made in the book and link this material to the second volume on families in catastrophe. References are combined at the end of the volume.

Chapter 1, by Hamilton I. McCubbin and Joan M. Patterson, lays the necessary theoretical groundwork for understanding the family stress and coping process. The authors review previous attempts to conceptualize family stress, especially the work of Hill and his ABCX Model of family crisis. They point out the complexities of this area of inquiry and the difficulties of identifying and classifying such concepts as stressor, hardship, demands, impact, and intensity. They argue persuasively that normative family transitions are important and often overlooked sources of stress. In an effort to systematically extend the work of Hill and others, the authors present their Double ABCX Model of family adaptation, which more fully accounts for post-crisis family reactions. Their model of family adjustment and adaptation is critical reading for the reader interested in understanding the complexity and significance of the chapters to follow.

In Chapter 2, Pauline G. Boss studies the stressors associated with change and development within the marital relationship over the life cycle. She applies the concept of boundary ambiguity, for which she is widely recognized, within the family stress framework. She notes that, for most marriages, mates' perceptions of boundaries and roles change dramatically but predictably over time and require the couple to adjust to these changes. Specific sources of stress for the married pair which are identified include (a) changes in expectations of each other; (b) changes in couple roles (e.g., homemaker to co-breadwinner); and (c) changes in demands. The last section is especially rich in implications for clinical intervention methods to facilitate marital coping.

Chapter 3, by Kaye L. Zuengler and Gerhard Neubeck, is a comprehensive overview of how sexuality can be a source of stress in families throughout the life cycle. They note, for example, that conspicuous silence, over-cautiousness, sexism, children's growing awareness of their bodies, pregnancy, and sexual dysfunction are normative but real sources of stress within the family. They note that open communication, as well as education about sexuality, is important in preventing serious stress.

In Chapter 4, Brent C. Miller and Judith A. Myers-Walls consider the stress associated with two significant family transitions: entering and exiting active parenthood. Sources of stress include abrupt increases in caregiving demands after birth and the gradual reduction as children leave home; psychological stressors over the welfare of the child; sense of accomplishment or failure as a parent; financial strain; and the sense of sacrifice of personal or marital growth for the sake of the children. The authors note that family and friends are vital social resources for parents in these transition points. A rich egalitarian parental relationship which includes consensus over various and shifting role reponsibilities is also important. They note that general parent education and support groups are also effective methods of coping.

Chapter 5, by Jeannie Kidwell, Judith L. Fischer, Richard M. Dunham, and Marc Baranowski, is also about parenthood, specifically about parenting a teenager. They examine in detail the developmental changes in both adolescents and their parents and note that the interaction of these developmental changes can make this an especially stressful transition. They view coping from a family systems perspective and outline the various ways a family can respond to the challenges of raising an adolescent child.

In Chapter 6, Denise A. Skinner, focuses on what recent statistics show to be a growing family lifestyle: the dual-career family. The dual-career family life cycle patterns differ from the traditional family, and the stressors and strains are different as well, including, for example, role overload and sex-role strain. Skinner suggests concrete coping strategies that these families use, such as making compromises or managing time carefully.

Constance Ahrons in Chapter 7 focuses on another "normative" phenomenon in contemporary America: divorce. So many families experience divorce today that Ahrons emphasises the importance of normalizing the event by seeing it as another kind of family change or transition, not as a sign of sickness or catastrophe. She puts forward the concept of the binuclear family to indicate two households including both parents even though they live apart. She outlines five stages of the divorce process, beginning with the individual awareness by one of the marital partners that something is wrong with the marriage, moving through trial separations, and ending with a redefinition of the family after the divorce. The latter portion of the chapter suggests ways in which those outside the family can help in the transition process: providing objective perspectives and education about the divorce process.

Chapter 8, by M. Janice Hogan, Cheryl Buehler, and Beatrice Robinson, is in some ways an extension of Chapter 7, because it is an examination of the post-divorce single-parent family. About 12 million children live in single-parent families in the U.S. Among the significant stressors of the single-parent family are a sense of loss and grief and the need to adapt to changes (e.g., child-centered issues, social sanctions, economic strains). The authors use a family management perspective to discuss stress-reducing behavior, such as setting appropriate goals, reorganizing routines, and redefining role expectations. Social support from outside the family is critical in supplementing these managerial efforts.

Chapter 9, by Emily and John Visher, also focuses on the post-marital transition, viewing the formation of a stepfamily as a stressful but normative life transition. In this chapter the authors identify five major sources of stress in terms of particular conditions which set stepfamilies apart from biological families: (a) members have experienced important losses; (b) members all come with past family histories; (c) parent-child bonds predate the new couple's relationship; (d) there is a biological parent elsewhere; and (e) the children are often members of two households. Successful coping strategies include having realistic expectations about stepfamily life, understanding the conflicting emotions children experience, and seeking support from outside the family. The authors conclude by alerting policymakers, counselors, and therapists of the need for greater awareness and understanding of stepfamily stress and proposing programs and policies to support this type of family.

Part II of this volume begins with a chapter by Gail F. Melson outlining some central concepts for understanding normative stress that is generated not by internal family transitions but by demands from outside the family. She first introduces Urie Bronfenbrenner's ecosystem model, "a nested series of interlocking environments," from the microsystems of family, work, friends, to the macrosystems of our political or economic structures. She argues convincingly that stress emerges as a result of a lack of fit between family and environmental demands, and that family adaptation is the achievement and maintenance of a relatively good fit. Thus, coping is viewed as an effort which allows the family some mastery over the environment in the process of reaching this proper fit. These concepts complement the definitions presented by McCubbin and Patterson in Chapter 1.

Chapter 11, by Joyce Portner, is about adult family members, the workplace, and how the demands of the workplace can conflict with demands of the family. Building on the groundwork laid by Skinner in Chapter 6, Portner discusses various patterns of work and family roles, and how the expectations that we have of ourselves, that society has of us, and that the employer has of us can generate stress. Portner advocates seeking a balance between work and family life and outlines both coping strategies internal to the family and assistance provided by the employer through policies such as flextime, parental leave time, childcare facilities, and educational programs.

In Chapter 12, Harriette P. McAdoo focuses on environmental stressors or racism as they affect the American Black family. The author uses the concept of "mundane extreme environmental stress" to underscore the normative but severe stress on minority families in America resulting from economic inequality, poor education, poor health care, inadequate housing, and other factors. But she also points out that the Black family is an enduring institution and an important source of support for Blacks. She notes that the reliance on extended family members among Blacks is greater than among whites; Black families traditionally also have more flexible role definitions for family members. Both of these are crucial in coping with omnipresent racism.

Raymond T. Coward and Robert T. Jackson focus on the stress of living in a rural environment in Chapter 13. The authors discuss the stress from economic and employment issues, community stressors, and geographic or climatic stressors. They suggest that rural life is far from the serene, tranquil stereotype that urban dwellers cherish. The authors say that there is little difference in both style and substance between rural and nonrural families: "mutual respect, cohesiveness, family history, personal values, open patterns of communication and emotional stability seem much more important than place of residence for predicting the ability to cope with stress." The authors would like to see greater attention paid to rural families and the stressors they must endure; they call for a comprehensive federal policy on rural America, improved health care and social services, and better information about rural families.

In Chapter 14, Mary Ann Noecker Guadagno studies the effect of the economic environment on families, specifically the effect of inflation.

After briefly defining inflation (increasing prices and decreasing value of money), and outlining some of its causes, she details how inflation affects families. She notes that inflation is hardest on poor families, who must spend a greater portion of their income on food, housing, gasoline, and other necessities that have been hit hard by inflationary pressures since the late 1960s. The hardships that inflation brings to families include limited access to education and advancement, involuntary moves, working extra hours for additional money, and so on. Resources important in coping include personal attributes (e.g., education, self-esteem, health), social support, and family flexibility. The author uses a family management framework to suggest coping strategies and advocates educational and counseling programs to prevent serious financial problems.

The final chapter, by the editors, provides both a synthesis of this first volume, and a bridge to Volume II, on Coping with Catastrophe. Family reactions to stress are remarkably similar, whether or not a normative or catastrophic change is the stressor. Moreover, these two sources of stress rarely operate in isolation from the other—victims of a tornado are part of families coping with childrearing or financial problems and nearly every family is touched by a catastrophe at some point in the life cycle. It is important to understand both kinds of stress, how they differ, and how families successfully support their members in dealing with stress.

PART

I

FAMILY TRANSITIONS

CHAPTER

1

Family Transitions:
Adaptation to Stress

HAMILTON I. McCUBBIN and
JOAN M. PATTERSON

John Sr. and Nancy Wilson became new parents two months ago. It has been difficult for, them. Nancy gave up a good paying job which she had had for eight years and John Sr. has taken on a second job to help pay the sudden increase in expenses. John and Nancy argue a lot over seemingly "minor" issues. Somehow, having a baby is more difficult than they expected; they aren't able to go out as a couple as much as they did before and Nancy is angry much of the time. So many things have happened to them in such a short period of time.

Their neighbor, Janet Lawrence, is recently divorced and has a five-year-old son; she is a single parent. Janet struggles with going back to work, finding quality child-care, and adjusting to this new neighborhood. While lonely and depressed some of the time, Janet is

This project was funded by a grant from the Agricultural Experiment Station, University of Minnesota. The authors would like to thank Dr. Richard Sauer, Director, Agricultural Experiment Station, and Dean Keith McFarland, College of Home Economics, for their support.

optimistic about the future. She is pleased with her job, excited about raising her son, and confident that despite some setbacks, she will be able to make a wonderful home for herself and her son.

Both of these families are under stress. However, they approach the difficult situation in different ways. Despite the very positive relationship between John and Nancy before the birth of their son, John Jr., the marital relationship is now strained and they are having difficulty coping. Janet, a single parent, struggles with the transition to being alone and a sole parent but maintains a very positive appraisal and outlook. Why the differences?

Family scholars have struggled with this very basic question with the hope of uncovering why some families are able to cope with ease and may even thrive on life's hardships, while other families, faced with similar if not identical stressors or family transitions, give up in the face of seemingly minor life changes. The purpose of this chapter is to introduce the reader to the ABCX and Double ABCX Models of family stress, which provide the major frameworks for understanding the chapters in *Stress and the Family*. These major theories and others (systems theory, family developmental theory, and Erik Erikson's psychosocial theory of individual development), as well as related research, can help us begin to explain why families differ in their definition and response to family transitions, the basic coping strategies they use, and the basic processes involved in family adaptation to stress and family crises.

THE HILL ABCX CRISIS MODEL REDEFINED

The earliest conceptual foundation for research to examine the variability in families was the Hill (1949, 1958) ABCX family crisis model:

A (the stressor event)—interacting with B (the family's crisis meeting resources)—interacting with C (the definition the family makes of the event)—produce X (the crisis) . . . (1958, p. 141).

Stressor and Hardships: Demands (a Factor)

The ABCX Model emerged from the field of sociology. Physiologists (Selye, 1974) in the field of medicine and psychologists (Lazarus, 1966; Mikhail, 1981) have also studied stress and coping. In an effort to integrate these lines of research, McCubbin and Patterson (1982) have defined a stressor as a life event (e.g., death, purchase of a home, parenthood, etc.) impacting upon the family unit which produces, or has the potential of producing, change in the family social system. This change may be in various areas of family life, such as its boundaries, goals, patterns of interaction, or values. Also part of the a factor are family hardships, which are defined as those demands on the family unit specifically associated with the stressor event. Examples of family hardships would be the additional expenses of raising John Jr. created by the stressor of the Wilson family's transition to parenthood. Predictably, Janet Lawrence's becoming the breadwinner after her divorce is a hardship created by the transition to single parenthood.

Classifying Stressors. Several family theorists have developed classification schemes for stressful life events and transitions. Hill (1958) classified stressors in terms of their impact upon the family unit:

1) Accession—changed family structure by adding a member (e.g., birth of a child)
2) Dismemberment—changed family structure by losing a member (e.g., death of a child)
3) Loss of family morale and unity (e.g., alcoholism, substance abuse)
4) Changed structure and morale (e.g., desertion, divorce).

In contrast, Lipman-Blumen (1975) advanced a comprehensive scheme for the assessment of family crises. Eight of her ten criteria appear to have direct application in the classification of stressors and in the determination of their impact on the family system:

1) Is the origin of the stressor from within the family system (e.g., mother goes back to work) or from outside the family (e.g., loss of a job)?
2) Does the impact of the stressor extend directly to all family members (e.g., divorce) or to only some members (e.g., adolescent has argument with friend)?
3) Is the onset of the stressor very sudden (e.g., tornado) or does it emerge gradually (e.g., pregnancy)?
4) Is the degree of severity of the stressor intense (e.g., a death) or mild (e.g., purchase of a new car)?
5) Is the length of adjustment to the stressor short-term (e.g., child starts school) or long-term (e.g., parent gets cancer)?

6) Can the stressor be expected (e.g., child becoming an adolescent) or does it occur unpredictably at random (e.g., an auto accident)?

7) Does the stressor emerge through natural causes (e.g., a hurricane) or as a result of artificial, human-made situations (e.g., loss of a job from increased use of technology)?

8) Does the family believe the stressor is one that can be solved (e.g., adjusting to a new home) or is it beyond control (e.g., inflation's effect on family finances)?

Some family scholars have followed the line of research conducted in psychosomatic medicine, investigating the links between stress and physical illness (Dohrenwend & Dohrenwend, 1974; Holmes & Rahe, 1967). Others have classified stressor events according to their desirability, frequency, and intensity. Pearlin and his associates (Menaghan, 1982; Pearlin & Schooler, 1978) have recorded the intensity of various life events by inquiring about family perceptions of "being bothered, unhappy, having problems coping," in order to arrive at strain scores. Investigators associated with the Family Stress and Coping Project of the University of Minnesota (McCubbin, Patterson, Bauman, & Harris, 1981; McCubbin, Patterson, & Wilson, 1981) have attempted to develop and test standardized scores (assigned by family members) for family life transitions such as marital strains, childbearing strains, financial strains, work transitions and strains, and illness strains.

Normative Intrafamily Transitions

The chapters presented in the first section of this book give systematic attention to normative events and transitions which evolve in the context of the family life cycle: marriage, parenthood, adolescence, dual career family, divorce, single-parent family, and stepfamily. One kind of research on these transitions addresses single "typical" or normative family transitions, such as transition to parenthood and retirement. Such events are viewed by family scholars as normative because they are ubiquitous (they occur to most families), expectable (families could anticipate their occurrence at certain scheduled points in the family life cycle), and short-term (not chronic). Generally, investigators have questioned subjects who have recently experienced a normative transition regarding the degree of adjustment and role change associated with the event and the importance of the transition.

Pearlin and associates (Menaghan, 1982; Pearlin & Schooler, 1978) have identified 13 or more changes in major roles related to marriage, occupation, and parenthood which are normative in that they are expectable, scheduled changes involving entrances into and exits from social roles as a consequence of movement through the life cycle. In their research, family members involved in normative role changes were assessed for their overall intensity of feelings regarding strain within roles. By and large, these investigators found that strain scores related to the experience of normative events were lower than scores for nonnormative events (e.g., catastrophic events as discussed in Volume II).

Family sociologists in the area of family development have focused on "critical role transitions" (Hill & Joy, 1979) which occur in most families and serve as demarcation points for stages in the family life cycle. "Normative," for these investigators, is associated with major developmental role changes and task assignment changes which occur in families with children. These normative stressor events are viewed as short-term experiences, accompanied by changes in role expectations and rules for interacting which occur during each transition period (e.g., parenthood, adolescence, dual careers). Thus, the amount of stress associated with each transition is related to the number or degree of role behavior changes for the whole family unit independent of any family perception of stress. To date, most of this work has been theoretical in nature, although some work has been done indicating that acquisition of roles is more stressful than loss of roles (George, 1980; Neugarten & Hagestad, 1977). This volume attempts to advance our understanding of the nature of transitional stress and how families cope and adapt to these transitions.

Resources (b Factor)

The b factor, the family's resources for meeting the demands of stressor events and hardships, has been described as the family's ability to prevent an event or a transition in the family from creating a crisis or disruption (Burr, 1973). Resources, then, become part of the family's capabilities for resisting crisis. Angell (1936), one of the early family theorists, attempted to describe more specifically what constituted family resources, emphasizing the value of family integration and family adaptability. Family integration refers to the bonds of coherence and unity running through family life, of which common interests, affection, and a sense of economic interdependence are perhaps the most prominent.

Family adaptability refers to the family's capacity to meet obstacles and shift its course of action. Cavan and Ranck (1938) and Koos (1946) identified additional resources: family agreement about its role structure; subordination of personal ambitions to family goals; satisfactions within the family obtained because it is successfully meeting the physical and emotional needs of its members; and goals toward which the family is moving collectively.

Family Definition: Focus on Stressor (c Factor)

The c factor in the ABCX Model is the definition the family makes of the seriousness of the experienced stressor. There are objective cultural definitions of the seriousness of life events and transitions which represent the collective judgment of the community. The c factor, however, is the family's subjective definition of the stressor, accompanying hardships, and their effect on the family. This subjective meaning reflects the family's values and previous experience in dealing with change and meeting crises. A family's outlook can vary from seeing life changes and transitions as challenges to be met to interpreting a stressor as uncontrollable and a prelude to the family's demise.

Family Tension: Stress and Distress

Stressor events, transitions, and related hardships produce tension which calls for management (Antonovsky, 1979). When this tension is not overcome, stress emerges. Family stress (as distinct from stressor) is defined as a state which arises from an actual or perceived imbalance between demand (e.g., challenge, threat) and capability (e.g., resources, coping) in the family's functioning. It is characterized by a nonspecific demand for adjustment or adaptive behavior. When this imbalance is due to demands exceeding resources, this is a state of hyperstress; conversely, when the imbalance is due to resources exceeding demands, the family experiences hypostress. In other words, stress varies depending upon the nature of the situation, the characteristics of the family unit, and the psychological and physical well-being of its members. Concomitantly, family distress is a negative state which results from the family's defining the demands-resources imbalance as unpleasant; eustress is a positive state which results from the family's defining the demands-resources imbalance as desirable, as a challenge family members enjoy.

Family Crisis: Demand for Change (x Factor)

Crisis (the x factor) has been conceptualized as a continuous variable denoting the amount of disruptiveness, disorganization, or incapacitation in the family social system (Burr, 1973). As distinct from stress, which is a demand-capability imbalance, crisis is characterized by the family's inability to restore stability and the constant pressure to make changes in the family structure and patterns of interaction. In other words, stress may never reach crisis proportions if the family is able to use existing resources and define the situation so as to resist change within the family system.

THE DOUBLE ABCX MODEL: FAMILY ADAPTATION

The original ABCX Model focused primarily upon pre-crisis variables that account for differences in family capability to cope with the impact of a stressor event and transition and that determine whether and to what degree the outcome is a crisis for the family. Assessing family post-crisis behavior requires a more dynamic model that focuses upon family efforts over time to recover from a crisis situation, i.e., family resiliency. The Double ABCX Model, which emerged from studies of war-induced family crises (McCubbin, Boss, Wilson, & Lester, 1980; McCubbin & Patterson, 1981, 1982, 1983), expands upon Hill's original ABCX Model and adds post-crisis variables in an effort to describe: (a) the additional life stressors and changes which may influence the family's ability to achieve adaptation; (b) the critical psychological and social factors families call upon and use in managing crisis situations; (c) the processes families engage in to achieve satisfactory resolution; and (d) the outcome of these family efforts. This Double ABCX Model is diagrammed in Figure 1.

Family Adaptation (xX Factor)

There are three units of analysis in the Double ABCX Model: (a) the individual family member, (b) the family unit, and (c) the community of which family members and the family unit are a part. Each of these units is characterized by both demands and capabilities. Family adaptation is achieved through reciprocal relationships, where the demands

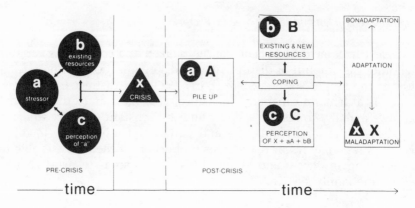

Figure 1. The Double ABCX Model

of one of these units are met by the capabilities at another, so as to achieve a "balance" simultaneously at two primary levels of interaction.

At the first level, a balance is sought between individual family members and the family unit (e.g., family encourages and supports adolescent needs for independence and adolescent family member completes family maintenance tasks, such as cleaning up the bedroom, or participates in shared family activities). Family stress or distress may emerge where there is a demand-capability imbalance at this level of family functioning. Specifically, the demands an individual member may place on the family may exceed the family's capability of meeting those demands, thus resulting in an imbalance. For example, John Sr.'s overcommitment to work to make financial ends meet has contributed to family imbalance, since Nancy's emotional needs are not adequately met. Therefore, the family is called upon to reconcile this matter and work to achieve a new balance between Nancy's demands and needs and the family unit. A balance might be achieved with greater ease if Nancy returned to work and John Sr. assumed more of the parenting role.

At the second level, a balance is sought between the family unit and the community of which this family is a part. It has frequently been observed that two social institutions, the family and the work community, compete for the involvement and commitment of family members, which often results in stress—a demand-capability imbalance at this second level of functioning. For example, the stressor of being the sole breadwinner in her family places Janet Lawrence in a potentially difficult situation. Janet's returning to work may precipitate an imbalance if the family demands (child-care needs, grandparent and parental pressures for her to stay home with her son) increase. Additionally, illnesses and a temporary breakdown in child-care arrangements may induce guilt and the felt need to fulfill home and work responsibilities with equal competence—to be "superwoman." The Lawrence family may be called upon to re-establish and maintain a balance between work-community demands and family life.

Therefore, family adaptation becomes the central concept in the Double ABCX Model used to describe the outcome of family efforts to achieve a new level of balance after a family crisis. In crisis situations, the family unit struggles to achieve a balance at both the individual-family and the family-community levels of family functioning. Since the family is a social system and a change in one level affects the other, family efforts at adaptation always simultaneously involve attentiveness and responsiveness to both levels of family functioning.

The concept of family adaptation is used to describe a continuum of outcomes reflecting family efforts to achieve a balance in functioning. The positive end of the continuum is called bonadaptation, and the negative end of the continuum is maladaptation. In Figure 2, the critical components of individual-to-family and family-to-community fit are outlined for each end of the adaptation continuum.

In their efforts to understand family post-crisis behavior social and behavioral scientists have tried to determine what specific dimensions of family life are likely to shape the course of family adjustment and adaptation over time. Two of the major factors from the Double ABCX are particularly relevant: family demands and family adaptive resources.

Family Demands: Pile-Up (aA Factor)

The demands or needs of individuals, families, and society are not static but change over time. For example, normative growth and de-

MALADAPTATION ———————	BONADAPTATION
deterioration in family integrity	family integrity strong
individual development curtailed	member development enhanced
family unit development curtailed	family unit development enhanced
loss of family independence and autonomy	family independence and control of environmental influence

Figure 2. Range of outcomes of family efforts to balance functioning.

velopment of individual adult members in the family (see Chapter 6 on dual careers), birth and development of children (see Chapters 4 and 5 on changes in children and adolescents), and changes in society (e.g., changing roles of women, declining birthrate, increasing number of divorces) are all demands which call for family adjustment and adaptation, and hence are sources of additional demands on the family unit. Because family crises evolve and are resolved over a period of time, families seldom are dealing with a single stressor. Rather, our studies suggest they experience a pile-up of demands, particularly from a chronic stressor such as caring for a disabled family member or in the aftermath of a major stressor, such as a death, a major role change for one member, or a natural disaster. This pile-up is referred to as the "aA" factor in the Double ABCX Model (see Figure 1).

There appear to be at least five broad types of stressors and strains contributing to a pile-up in the family system in a crisis situation: (a) the initial stressor and its hardships; (b) normative transitions; (c) prior strains; (d) the consequences of family efforts to cope; and (e) ambiguity, both intrafamily and social.

Stressor and Its Hardships. Inherent in the occurrence of a stressful event such as the addition of a new member to the family unit, a divorce, or a member going back into the work force, are specific hardships which increase and possibly intensify the difficulties families face. Certainly, in the case of John and Nancy Wilson, the hardships of giving up a job (Nancy), picking up an additional job (John Sr.), and the infant-caring tasks contributed to pile-up. Janet Lawrence also struggled with a pile-up due to the hardships of returning to the work force, raising a child alone, and relocating to get a new start for her family.

Normative Transitions. Even though the Wilson and Lawrence families faced the stressor of a major transition (parenthood and divorce, respectively), they also faced the potential of additional stressors or transitions. For example, these families experienced the normal growth and development of child members (e.g., increasing need for nurturance and supervision; increasing need for independence), of adult members (e.g., spouse's desire to continue with her career; mother's increasing need for a meaningful relationship), of the extended family (e.g., illness and death of grandparents), and family life cycle changes (e.g., children entering school, adolescence). Such transitions occur at the same time, but often quite independent of the initial stressor. These demands or opportunities place additional demands upon the family unit, since they also call for family adjustment and adaptation.

Prior Strains. It would appear that most family systems carry with them some residue of strain, which may be the result of unresolved hardships from earlier stressors or transitions or may be inherent in ongoing roles such as parent or employer (Pearlin & Schooler, 1978). When a new stressor is experienced by the family, these prior strains are exacerbated and families become aware of them as demands in and of themselves. For example, Nancy and John Sr. struggle with the prior strain of Nancy's loss of status and esteem as a result of her giving up an important job which she valued. Surely, Janet Lawrence struggles with the unresolved strain of her prior marriage, much of which will take a considerable amount of time to resolve. These prior strains contribute to the pile-up of difficulties both of these families now face. These prior strains are not usually discrete events which can be identified as occurring at a specific point in time; rather, they emerge more insidiously in the family. They do, however, contribute to the pile-up of demands families must contend with in a crisis situation.

Consequences of Family Efforts to Cope. The fourth source of pile-up includes stressors and strains which emerge from specific behaviors the family may use in an effort to cope with the crisis situation. For example, John Sr. attempted to deal with increased expenses by assuming another job. Coping by getting a second job became another source of family strain, contributing to Nancy's loneliness and frustration. Janet Lawrence's decision to move to a new community also created another source of strain; meeting new friends, fitting in, and establishing a credit record were additional demands for the Lawrence family.

Intrafamily and Social Ambiguity. A certain amount of ambiguity is inherent in every stressor, since change produces uncertainty about the future. Internally, the family may experience ambiguity about its structure; is Janet Lawrence's former spouse (Bill) still a member of the family because he is Todd's (five-year-old boy) father? What about Todd's paternal grandparents? Are they part of the family system? Boss (1977, 1980) has suggested that boundary ambiguity within the family system is a major stressor, since a system needs to be sure of its components, that is, who is inside of the system boundaries, physically and psychologically, and who is outside.

Additionally, given the expectation that society will offer guidelines or blueprints for families coping with crises, it is probable that families will face the added strain of social ambiguity in those situations where needed social prescriptions for crisis resolution are unclear or absent (McCubbin & Patterson, 1982). For example, Janet Lawrence also faced the stigma and loss of status associated with a divorce. Society's efforts to normalize this major transition (see Chapter 7) are important in easing family strains. The family's ability to manage stress may depend upon the efficacy and/or adequacy of the solutions the culture or community provide. However, these community solutions may lag far behind the times and offer little to families struggling to manage a difficult situation.

Family Adaptive Resources (bB Factor)

Resources are part of the family's capabilities for meeting demands and needs which emerge in the context of a crisis. Three kinds of resources affecting a family's adaptation to crises are: (a) family members' personal resources; (b) the family system's internal resources; and (c) social support.

Personal resources refer to the broad range of characteristics of individual family members which are potentially available to any family member in times of crisis. When members have sufficient appropriate resources, they are less likely to view a crisis situation as problematic. There are four basic components of personal resources: financial (economic well-being), education (contributing to cognitive ability that facilitates realistic stress perception and problem-solving skills), health (physical and emotional well-being), and psychological resources (personality characteristics) (George, 1980; Lazarus, 1966). Pearlin and Schooler (1978) have identified two personal psychological resources residing within the self which can reduce the stressful consequences of social strain: (a) self-esteem—the positiveness of one's attitude toward one's self; and (b) mastery—the extent to which one perceives control over one's life chances in contrast to being fatalistically ruled.

Family system resources gained prominence in both Hill's original formulations of the b factor and in Burr's (1973) synthesis of the research literature. One promising conceptualization of family resources in the management of crisis has evolved out of Pratt's (1976) analysis of family health behavior. Pratt has described the "energized family" as being endowed with a fluid internal organization characterized by flexible role relationships and shared power; this organization promotes personal growth and member autonomy.

Family cohesion (or integration) and adaptability (Olson, Russell, & Sprenkle, 1979; Olson, Sprenkle, & Russell, 1979; Sprenkle & Olson, 1978) appear to be two of the most important family resources in the management of crises. Olson and McCubbin (1982) advanced the hypothesis that families functioning moderately along the dimensions of cohesion and adaptability are likely to make a more successful adaptation to crises. Too much cohesion can create enmeshment and too much adaptability is chaotic for the family system. Conversely, too little cohesion leads to disengagement of family members and too little adaptability results in a rigid family system.

Social support offers families information at an interpersonal level which provides (a) emotional support, leading the members or family unit to believe that they are cared for and loved; (b) esteem support, leading the members or family unit to believe they are esteemed and valued; and (c) network support, leading the members or family unit to believe that they belong to a network involving mutual obligation and mutual understanding (Cobb, 1976). Granovetter (1973) has referred to social support as information disseminated with regard to problem-solving and new social contacts for help.

Both the availability of social networks (e.g., neighbors, kinship groups, and mutual self-help groups) and the ability of such networks to provide support have been found to vary greatly (see Chapter 12). Many have noted that the elderly are particularly likely to have low social network involvement due to lack of money, loss of family and friends, and lack of transportation (Lee, 1979). Lower-class families have been found to give support in the form of services, in contrast to middle-class families who are more likely to give gifts or loans (Lee, 1979; Troll, 1971). Litwak and Szelenyi (1969) found that neighbors and friends provide an important source of assistance for short-term problems, such as one-day illnesses or temporary child-care. Ethnic and minority families have made extensive use of extended family support (Lin, Simeone, Ensel, & Kuo, 1979; Lopata, 1978)

Intergenerational supports continue as children leave home and establish families of their own. Troll (1971) and Sussman (1976) have concluded that most older persons maintain close, viable, and satisfying relationships with their adult children. In addition, most older and younger family members report satisfaction with the frequency and quality of intergenerational relationships. This pattern of frequent and satisfying interaction among generations of adult family members living in independent households has been referred to by Hill (1970) as a modified extended family system. When all three generations, older, middle and younger, are involved in patterns of support and resource exchange, they have some protection against the harmful effects of stress and crises.

Mutual self-help groups have been defined as associations of individuals or family units who share the same problem, predicament, or situation and band together for the purpose of mutual aid. Mutual help groups, in addition to being supportive of their members, are also action-oriented, often focusing upon changing attitudes and policies which affect their problem situation (Katz, 1970; Lieberman, Berman, & Associates, 1979; McCubbin, 1979).

In general, social support serves as a protector against the effects of stressors and promotes recovery from stress or crises experienced in the family. Research has revealed the influence of social support as a protective factor against the complications of pregnancy and childbirth (Nuckolls, Kassel, & Kaplan, 1972) and in promoting medical compliance (Baekland & Lundwall, 1975). Investigators have indicated that social support makes individuals and family units less vulnerable to crises when they experience stressors such as job terminations or difficult work environments (Gore, 1978), or natural disasters such as floods (Erickson, 1976) or tornados (Drabeck, Key, Erickson, & Kaplan, 1975). The role of social support in promoting the family's recovery from crises has been indicated in the case of psychiatric illness (Caplan, 1974; Eaton, 1978), death (Parkes, 1972), divorce (Colletta, 1979), and multiproblem families (Burns & Freedman, 1976).

Family Definition and Meaning (cC Factor)

In the Double ABCX Model, the cC factor is family definition and meaning. Specifically, in the face of crises and the demand for changes in the family unit, the family unit struggles to give new "meaning" to the situation. When families are able to redefine the situation and give it new meaning (i.e., purpose, value, understanding and direction), it works to (a) clarify the issues, hardships, and tasks so as to render them more manageable and responsive to problem-solving efforts; (b) decrease the intensity of the emotional burdens associated with the crisis situation; and (c) encourage the family unit to carry on with its fundamental tasks of promoting members' social and emotional development. Generally, family efforts to redefine a situation as a "challenge," an "opportunity for growth," or to endow the crisis with a special meaning, such as "believing that it is the best for everyone," appear to facilitate family coping and adaptation. Viewed in this way, the family's definition and meaning, the cC factor, form a critical component of family coping. Janet Lawrence, the single parent, tried to look favorably upon the difficult transition in which she was involved. It would appear that Janet defined her hardships as "challenges" and a "chance to build a new life for herself and son." This positive appraisal would be helpful to her efforts to establish a professional career and to endure future hardships. Positive definitions which facilitate adaptive coping do not include a "Pollyanna" attitude of minimizing what is needed or a denial of the reality of the situation, both of which could hinder successful adjustment and adaptation.

THE FAMILY PROCESS OF ADJUSTMENT AND ADAPTATION

The processes of family adjustment and adaptation, called the *family adjustment and adaptation response* (FAAR) (McCubbin & Patterson, 1983) are presented in Figure 3. These processes, which families use to achieve stability in the face of stressful normative and nonnormative life events and transitions, are best viewed as two distinct phases: the adjustment phase in response to a stressor and the adaptation phase which occurs following a family crisis.

The Family Adjustment Phase

It is assumed that in the period of time preceding a stressor event or transition, family functioning is relatively stable. However, this stability does not preclude the possibility of some disturbing patterns of family interaction (e.g., marital conflict, sibling conflict, parent-child conflict). So, in reality, the family could be anywhere along the adaptation continuum from bonadaptation to maladaptation. Where a family is along the continuum of adaptation influences its vulnerability to the impact of a subsequent stressor event or transition, but the important characteristic of the family before the impact of a stressor event or transition is the general sense of satisfaction and stability about the family structure and patterns of interaction.

When a family initiates or is confronted with a stressor or transition, it experiences a cluster of demands which include (a) the stressor event or transition; (b) the hardships directly associated with this situation; and (c) prior strains already existing in the family system which may be exacerbated by the transition and hence come into the awareness of one

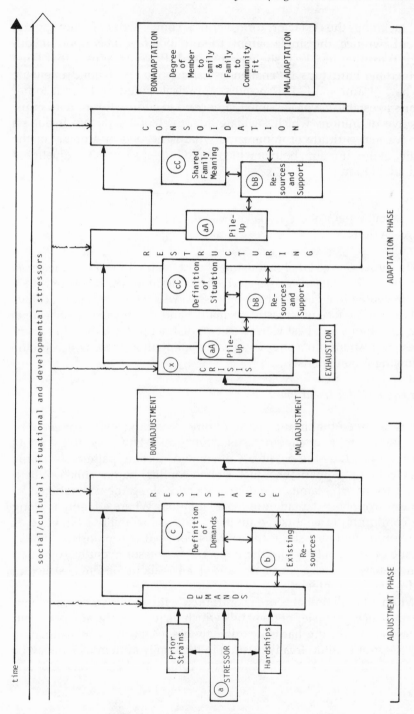

Figure 3. F A A R—Family Adjustment and Adaptation Response

or more of its members. In the usual course of action, the family attempts to make adjustments in its pattern of interaction, with minimal change or disruption of the family's established patterns of behavior and structure. These efforts can best be described as family resistance to change. During this phase the family makes an effort to protect itself from change by maintaining its established patterns. For example, the Wilson family made every effort to keep things as they were (e.g., going out, spending time together) before John Jr. was born. They tried to maintain aspects of their previous lifestyle when there was more money from Nancy's income.

Adjustment Coping Strategies. A family may employ at least three basic adjustment coping strategies, used alone or in combination to bring about family adjustment: avoidance, elimination, and assimilation. Avoidance can be defined as family efforts to deny or ignore the stressor and other demands in the belief and hope that they will go away or resolve themselves. Elimination is an active effort by the family to rid itself of all demands by changing or removing the stressor, or altering the definition of the stressor. Both avoidance and elimination responses serve to minimize or protect the family unit from having to make modifications in the family's structure. Assimilation, the third adjustment coping strategy, involves family efforts to accept the demands created by the stressor into its existing structure and patterns of interaction. The family absorbs the demands by making only minor changes within the family unit. John Sr. and Nancy first tried to maintain their old patterns by treating John Jr.'s arrival as "expected and routine" (that is, until little John's needs required that the Wilson family reconsider the situation; expenses were higher and John Jr. needed a fulltime caretaker). Very little change is made, for the family unit has an adequate and appropriate supply of existing resources which may be employed or reallocated. This supply of resources influences the family's definition and appraisal of demands, as well as which coping strategies are used. For example, if the Wilson family had had sufficient income to acquire a full-time baby-sitter, and had felt comfortable with such an arrangement, their definition and coping strategies might very well have been different.

Adjustment can be viewed as a short-term response by families, adequate to manage many family life changes, transitions, and demands. However, there are occasions when adjustment-oriented coping strategies are insufficient to meet the demands to which families are exposed. These situations are likely to emerge in those circumstances in which

(a) the nature of the stressor or transition involves a structural change in the family system (e.g., parenthood, divorce); (b) the nature, number, and duration of demands depletes the family's existing resources (e.g., financial savings spent); (c) the number and persistence of prior unresolved strains also tax the family's resources (e.g., continued conflict with prior spouse); (d) the family's capabilities and resources are basically inadequate or underdeveloped to meet the demands (e.g., insufficient income to meet child-care demands or to be a single parent); and (e) the family overtly or covertly seizes the opportunity to produce structural changes in the family unit by allowing or facilitating a demand-capability imbalance or family crisis (e.g., allowing unresolved marital conflict to continue as a prelude to dissolution of a marriage). Consequently, as the demand-capability imbalance persists and possibly increases, a family moves toward or into a state of crisis.

Crisis, as already defined, involves disorganization and the demand for changes in the family unit to restore stability at its prior level or another (higher or lower) level of family functioning. This movement to initiate change in the family unit marks the beginning of the adaptation phase of the family adjustment and adaptation response. It is very important to note that a family "in crisis" does not carry the stigmatizing value judgment that somehow the family has failed, is dysfunctional, or in need of professional counseling. Rather, many family crises are normative and involve changes in family structure and established patterns of interaction in order to cope with developmental changes in family members and the family system. Other family crises are actively set in motion by family decisions to make structural changes (e.g., separation, dual career, reentry into the work force) or shifts in core family values or goals as a planned step to improve family conditions, reduce financial or emotional strains, and enhance the overall functioning of the family unit.

The Family Adaptation Phase

Families in crisis, which face excessive demands and depleted resources, come to realize that in order to restore some functional stability and/or improve family satisfaction they need to restructure—make changes in their existing structure which may include modifications in established roles, rules, goals, and/or patterns of interaction. Additionally, after they have made these initial changes, the family members are called upon to make subsequent changes in an effort to consolidate—bring the entire family into a coherent unit working together around and in support of the newly instituted changes. These processes of restructuring and consolidation evolve over time as families work towards adaptation.

Adaptive Coping Strategies. Families often call upon social support to ease the strains of restructuring. Resources and support influence the family's transition through the restructuring phase by buffering the impact of pile-up (e.g., providing resources to resolve problems), by influencing the definition of the situation (e.g., positive appraisal, sense of mastery), and maximizing the solutions available (e.g., chance for a second job or chance for wife to return to prior job).

Family efforts at restructuring and consolidation are also facilitated by the adaptive coping strategies of synergizing, interfacing, and compromising.

Synergizing refers to family efforts to coordinate and pull together as a unit to accomplish a shared lifestyle and orientation which cannot be achieved by any member alone but only through mutuality and interdependence. Family members are attuned to each other as they work to synchronize and coordinate their respective perceptions, needs, and resources. For example, John and Nancy Wilson might have tried to synergize by having Nancy return to her valued job, with John sharing more directly in caring for their new baby.

Family efforts are not limited to internal changes in the family unit. Because the family is a semi-closed system with commitments to and transactions with other social institutions (e.g., work, school, community groups), the family also works at interfacing with the community to achieve a new "fit." The initial complementary relationship between the community and family life may be disturbed by the family's internal restructuring and therefore demand a new set of rules and transactions. Janet Lawrence, for example, sought to find a new beginning by relocating to a new community, and thus, as a single parent, was called upon to reestablish new fit within the community.

Families are seldom able to achieve perfect intrafamily and family-to-community fit where all needs are absolutely met. Predictably, successful consolidation and adaptation call for compromising through a realistic appraisal of the family's circumstances and a willingness to accept and lend support to a less than perfect resolution. For example, John Sr. and Nancy continue to struggle with their conflicts with the realization that they will need to work out a compromise.

Successful adaptation also requires coping efforts directed at system maintenance, i.e., integration, morale, and member self-esteem. As the family works to restructure and consolidate, it needs to know that there is something, i.e., the family itself, worth making all these changes for. It would appear that extended lack of attention to these needs of family members and the unit may be a major contributor to family breakdown.

Observations of family coping with transitions and nonnormative life events outside of the family unit reveal that the family strategies of coping are not created in a single instant and not directed at a single stressor. Because the family is a system, coping strategies involve the management of various dimensions of family life simultaneously: (a) maintaining satisfactory internal conditions for communication and family organization; (b) promoting member independence and self-esteem; (c) maintenance of family bonds of coherence and unity; (d) maintenance and development of social supports in transactions with the communty; and (e) maintenance of some efforts to control the impact of the demands and the amount of change in the family unit. Coping then becomes a process of achieving a balance in the family system which facilitates organization and unity and promotes individual growth and development.

CONCLUSIONS AND IMPLICATIONS

Family transitions over the life span predictably create stress and often move the family unit to a state of crisis. How well families negotiate and navigate their way through these critical transitions has and will continue to be a major concern and interest of family scholars, counselors, family life educators, and policymakers.

The observations and theoretical frameworks described in this chapter serve to sensitize as well as orient us to the complex ways and strategies families employ to cope with these predictable, yet demanding situations. But even more important, the research on family transitions as stressors serves to underscore the importance of family policies and programs directed at promoting family strengths and capabilities in order that families can successfully resolve these crises on their own. Furthermore, the research observations and theory-building efforts to date offer counselors and policymakers targets and goals around which interventions and programs can be built. For example, we have witnessed a growth in the number of programs directed at educating parents to cope with the transition to parenthood and with divorce. One of the unique aspects of these programs is the strong emphasis placed upon the development of support networks and groups through which families gain practical information, understanding, and a sense of self-worth.

As we move ahead with research and theory-building and seek to improve our understanding of family behavior in response to stress, we can anticipate a greater awareness of how and why families are able to endure very difficult transitions with such ease. Even more important, we can expect to improve our understanding of how family members, the family unit and the community work together to cope with stress. This chapter and the chapters to follow on family stress and coping are designed to foster this line of scientific inquiry and ultimately promote future efforts directed at supporting families under stress.

2

The Marital Relationship: Boundaries and Ambiguities

PAULINE G. BOSS

Esther had an unusually close relationship with her parents. When she and David decided to get married, Esther's mother helped plan the wedding down to the smallest detail; Esther didn't think of buying a piece of furniture without her mother's stamp of approval. Even after Esther and David had been married a few months, Esther called home every day and was quick to respond to her parents' needs. When she and David had a fight, she went to her parents' home for the night. David finally angrily told her, "Enough! Make up your mind which family you're in!"

After several stormy scenes, Esther decided to seek out the help of a therapist. She gradually came to see that she was really involved in two separate families, both competing for her loyalty and her presence. After time and some effort to strengthen her self-esteem, she was able to declare that her first loyalty was to herself as a woman and that her relationship with David came before her relationship with her parents. She saw herself as an equal partner with her husband.

Esther and David worked out the stress in their marriage. With the help of a therapist they clarified Esther's attitude toward her husband and her parents. The problems around this issue had to be resolved before the couple could deal with other problems in their lives; the ambiguity in their relationship had to be clarified first.

MARRIAGE AS A STRESSOR

Most couples would agree that the main sources of stress in their marriages are disagreements between the husband and wife over money or childrearing, sexual problems, or one partner's job demands. All of these issues and their effects on the married couple, as well as on other members of the family, are considered in detail in other chapters in this volume (cf. Chapters 3-5; 11). In this chapter, however, we will study the marital relationship itself: the "axis of the family system" (Satir, 1964, p. 1).

Almost 95% of Americans will get married at least once in their lifetimes, yet the high divorce rate in the U.S. today suggests that marital relationships are failing to satisfy the needs or expectations of many individuals. Some of the stressors of marriage will be considered here, using the concept of boundary ambiguity, the uncertainty about who is in the family system, when they are there, and what their roles are. This uncertainty can be about the boundary (1) between a spouse and his or her family of origin; (2) between the spouses themselves; or (3) as a result of family transitions over the life cycle. Coping with marital stress will be seen in terms of clarifying this ambiguity. Special attention will be paid to the role of the therapist or counselor in clarifying boundaries in the marital and family systems.

BOUNDARY AMBIGUITY AND STRESS IN MARRIAGE

In a marriage, the husband and wife share leadership of the family system. We define them as co-executives of the family system; they work together to meet the needs of the family and of each other. Meeting these needs includes providing material things, like food, clothing, and shelter, as well as providing love, esteem, and support to the children and any other family members, and to each other. The task of managing and directing this system can last as long as 50 or 60 years, or only for a few months.

Because co-executives must work together, it is imperative that they communicate frequently and clearly with one another, that they understand their tasks and their relationships with their own parents, with their children, with each other, and with the outside world. It is the thesis of this chapter that *one of the barriers to effective marital communication is confusion or uncertainty about any of these roles or relationships.* This uncertainty is called *boundary ambiguity.* The ambiguity is the stressor in the relationship, but the ambiguity may be about different issues; for example, the boundary between one spouse and his or her family of origin or between the spouses themselves could be unclear.

Boundary Ambiguity Defined

As with any living system, the family has a boundary or limit. Unlike the borders of a city or the walls of a cell, a family's walls or boundaries are difficult to determine. Family boundaries are indicated by who is performing what roles and tasks inside the family, and who is perceived by the family members, and especially by the executive pair, as being *present* inside the family. For example, parents can keep grown children inside the family boundary after they leave home, just as Esther's parents did. Esther complied by remaining loyal to her parents, fulfilling their every wish, and letting them make decisions for her. Boundaries in this case were set by roles, loyalties, and perceptions. When David demanded that Esther decide which family she was in, he was expressing his own perception of boundary ambiguity—was his wife in or out of their family? How far should her parents be allowed to infiltrate the boundaries of their family? This fuzziness about who is in and who is out has been characterized as boundary ambiguity (Boss, 1975, 1980a, 1980b) or diffuse boundaries (Minuchin, 1974).

Another example would be the husband who is physically present in the family but too busy or too preoccupied with work demands to talk to his wife on personal matters. He is what is called "physically present but psychologically absent" (Boss, 1975, 1977).

In contrast, during wartime, families often have to endure long periods without the husband at home. He may be overseas on a tour of duty or, worse, a POW or missing in action. In this case the husband is physically absent, but the family may behave as if he were there. A mother might say to her child, "Your father doesn't like that sort of behavior." He is *psychologically* present for the family members. In both these examples there is an incongruity between physical and psychological presence which creates a skewed perception of who is inside the family system's boundaries.

In David and Esther's marriage, Esther was psychologically absent although physically present. She was emotionally unavailable to her husband yet was highly present both emotionally and physically for her parents. David had a wife in the house, but she was not "there" for him. In other families one spouse may be highly involved with the children (physically and psychologically present) but "absent" for the mate (physically present but psychologically absent). Such ambiguity is a major source of stress in a marriage.

Boundary Ambiguity in the Family of Origin

Experiences in one's family of origin affect how one functions in marriage. Esther, for example, was still enmeshed in her parents' lives. She was continuing her childhood role of smoothing their troubled relationship. She was, in a way, a parent to her parents. The same role responsibilities that prevented her from being simply a daughter prevented her from feeling free of her parents to be a wife. The cross-generational ambiguity had to be resolved before she could establish a co-executive relationship in her own marriage.

Incest victims provide another example of how ambiguity between the generational systems can affect one's relationship with a mate. When a father crosses personal and generational boundaries to use his daughter sexually, she may have trouble in adulthood knowing her own sexual boundaries in relation to other men. She may marry a man who also invades her personal boundaries or she may build a wall so high and impenetrable around herself that no man can ever get to her again, psychologically or physically. Her confusion about her own individual boundaries, based on her incest experience, may affect her subsequent relationships with men.

Other kinds of family boundary issues affect individuals in marital relationships. Children of alcoholic family systems frequently bring to their marriages remnants of the survival behavior they learned. They may be pleasers, fixers, caretakers. They may avoid conflict at all cost because of their fear of the violence that surrounded them when they were children. In childhood they may have been the family executives, managing what their parents could or would not. For such children, generational boundaries were and still may be ambiguous. When they marry and try to establish a co-executive relationship with their spouses, they still may hunger for the nurturance and support they lacked when they were young. At the same time, they are used to being "in charge" and may resent a partner with whom they must now share family executive functions.

Marriage counselors and marital therapists are very familiar with this phenomenon of unclear boundaries between families of origin and the nuclear family. Too often, people marry before they have resolved ambiguities in their relationships to parents and while their sense of their own identity is still blurred. Indeed, they may choose partners and marry in order to work on this process of boundary clarification. Individuals make better choices in marriage partners if they first clarify boundary issues with the family of origin. This may be one of the reasons that those who marry very young have a higher divorce rate; it simply takes time and maturity for young people to accomplish psychological separation from their families of origin.

After marriage a boundary must be established and maintained between the nuclear family and the extended family system. Many couples agree that relationships with in-laws are a source of tension and difficulty in their marriages. The spouses must establish themselves, demonstrate that they can manage on their own, and take on the roles and tasks necessary to the management of their own family. For example, Esther eventually learned to turn to her husband, rather than her parents, for emotional support and joint decision-making.

Boundary Ambiguity between Marital Partners

Marital stress often revolves around boundary ambiguity between partners. Sex roles, idealistic expectations, and competition between spouses are three important areas of such ambiguity.

Sex Roles. Consider the example of a husband and wife who see the sex roles in marriage differently. When Mike and Nancy married, there was no disagreement about roles; they both believed that the man should have the final decision-making power in the family. But when Mike got a new job and had to travel a good deal, the clarity of roles and boundaries broke down. Mike still wanted to be in charge, but Nancy became more and more frustrated. She saw the need for immediate decisions on day-to-day matters about the house and the children: Could nine-year-old Tony stay overnight at his friend's house? Could Nancy get a much needed new vacuum cleaner at a one-day-only sale? Nancy certainly was capable of making such decisions, but felt guilty or afraid about Mike's reaction. Sometimes he laughed at her for being so hesitant about such simple things, but when she went ahead and bought a tricycle for their younger daughter, Mike was furious. Ambiguity about who makes decisions created stress for the family.

If this couple were to clarify the ambiguities in their co-executive system and to shift some of the decision-making responsibility to the wife, the change would challenge their traditional conceptions of the roles of men and women, of husbands and wives in families. Not only would it require them to clarify their perceptions, but it would also require them to change role assignments in the entire family system. This change would include the children, who may be modeling their parents, and the couple's own parents, who may not approve of a more equal role for the wife.

Idealistic Expectations. When Linda and Jerry were dating, Linda would imagine what their married life would be like. She wanted it to be perfect: The couple would be absolutely devoted to one another. They would spend every minute together, share interests, intuitively know what the other was thinking. Just like *True Romances!* But after they were married, this instant devotion somehow failed to happen. Jerry would go out after dinner about once a week to play baseball with his buddies. He seemed to be more interested in them than in Linda, or so she said to herself. Jerry did not seem to understand what she was upset about when she would complain about his evenings spent with friends. "You don't expect me to drop all my friends just because we are married, do you?" he would ask; but of course this was exactly what she did expect.

Both partners felt resentment and disappointment about the situation. The two had different expectations about what married life would be like, different ideas about how the boundary between the two of them was to be drawn. Linda's idealization of the marital relationship may have been unrealistic; she wanted the boundary between the two of them virtually to disappear. Jerry, on the other hand, saw himself as an individual with his own friends and his own interests and was not sensitive to Linda's expectations and emotional needs. The clash of expectations resulted in little or no agreement on where the boundaries in their marriage would be drawn. This was a stressor in their marriage which would require immediate attention. Marriage counselors may find their first task in helping couples like Linda and Jerry is to clarify these unspoken expectations and promises. The couple may be asked to draw up a written contract, where they can pin down and make explicit their values (Sager, 1976).

Competition. Mark and Michelle shared a great many interests. They were lawyers in a Western city. They had met in college and Mark's interest in the law had inspired Michelle to pursue that career herself. They both felt that their shared interests would be a good basis for their marriage. But when Mark was offered a position in a well-regarded law firm, Michelle was envious. He, in turn, resented the fact that she was asked to chair a committee of the local bar association. They enjoyed the fact that they belonged to a highly competitive profession, but were not able to prevent that competition from intruding on their married life.

The boundary ambiguity in this case relates to the relationship between themselves and their jobs. How could they clarify which behaviors and roles were appropriate to marriage and which to careers? Were they "there" for each other or so wrapped up in their work that they both were psychologically separate?

The Role of Perception. These three examples demonstrate the variety of situations where ambiguity or uncertainty can act as a stressor for married couples. It is important to realize, though, that the ambiguity was in the couples' *perception* of the situation.

An outside observer may have difficulty distinguishing ambiguities from clear boundaries in a marriage. For example, a husband and wife may appear to be separate from each other, to lead separate lives while sharing the same house. Before calling the situation an incongruity between physical and psychological presence, the observer must ask how the roles are perceived by each partner. While the partners seem to lead two separate lives, she caring for the children, he devoting himself to the job, and each having a great deal of individual freedom, they may be very clear that their sexual relationship is exclusive and their marital relationship harmonious. In such a family, the wife may indeed act as a "single parent" in rearing their children but knows her husband fills the role of confidant and lover. If they agree on how their roles are divided, there is no ambiguity in their relationship. What is important is how both perceive the boundaries of their relationship insofar as role performance is concerned. Ambiguity occurs when the two do not agree, and this is where stress can begin.

Boundary Ambiguity and Marital Stress Across the Life Cycle

As was noted in the Introduction to this volume, the marital and family life cycles involve many transitions as members join or leave the nuclear family system. Children are born and launched; couples are married and possibly divorced and remarried to others; family members die. These transitions are all potential stressors for the family, as many other chapters in this book make clear. They can also be seen in terms of the ambiguity they generate and the accompanying stress that is a consequence for the married couple.

Based on the perceptions of family therapists and developmental theorists and on initial testing of the boundary ambiguity concepts, one can propose that the greater the boundary ambiguity in the marital relationship at various developmental and normative junctures throughout the family life cycle, the higher the marital and individual stress and the greater risk for marital dysfunction. Resolution of the ambiguity is necessary before the couple can reorganize and move on toward new functioning at a lower level of stress. Non-resolution of the ambiguity holds the couple at a higher stress level by blocking the regenerative power to reorganize.

Obviously, some couples resolve the stress of family membership change more easily than do others. For example, marital roles may be quickly reassigned when a new baby joins a family. The father takes over the cooking; in-laws help with housework temporarily. Boundaries are maintained after the baby is born by a major shifting of roles and tasks within the family system. Furthermore, interactions of the family with the outside world may be altered. The wife may give up her job for a while to stay with the baby, which is a major boundary change for a woman used to daily interaction with the outside work world. If she chooses to go back to work, either for financial reasons or for her own self-esteem, and hires day-care help to care for the child, she may experience some uncertainty about her role in the family. She may need or want to work but feel she should be with her new baby. Or a father may feel closed out of his wife's emotional life by the new child; the baby may be satisfying her needs in a way that he has not. In these examples, the potential for family stress is great.

To emphasize the recurrence and complexity of such situations across time and to show how boundary ambiguities constantly affect the marriage, Table 1 presents some examples (with related research references) of boundary change over the life cycle. These boundary changes are a consequence of family members moving in and out of the family system.

COPING IN MARRIAGE

For the executives in a family system, coping combines individual and group strategies. The coping process must start with the recognition that something stressful has occurred. An emotional response must result from that recognition and some active or passive (fight or flight) behavior

TABLE 1
Selected References to Illustrate Normative Life-Span Boundary Changes

Type of Life-Span Family Boundary Changes	Boundary Stressors Related to Physical and Psychological Membership in the System
Formation of the dyad Rapoport (1963)	*acquisition of a mate *acquisition of in-laws *realignment with family of orientation *incorporating or rejecting former friendships
Birth of the first child LeMasters, 1957 Russell, 1974 Pridham, Hansen & Conrad, 1977	*acquisition of a new member *possible separation from extra-familial work world *if so, loss of working colleagues, etc.
Children first going to school Anderson, 1976 Klein & Ross, 1958	*separation of child from the family system to the world of school *acquisition of child's teacher, friends, and peers, i.e., acceptance of them as part of the child's world
Job-related parent/spouse absence or presence Hill, 1949 Boulding, 1950 Boss, 1975, 1980 McCubbin, et al., 1976 Boss, et al., 1979 Hooper, 1979	*fluctuating acquisition *and* separation due to extra-familial role, i.e., military service, routine absence of the corporate executive etc. Stress results from repeated exit and re-entry of the member. Also includes job changes such as return of mother to college or work after she's been a full-time homemaker or retirement of father from work back into the home.
Adolescent children leaving home Stierlin, 1974 Boss & Whitaker, 1979	*separation of adolescent from the family system to his peers, school or job system *acquisition of the adolescent's peers and intimates/same and opposite sex
Taking in child(ren) not your own or blending children from different dyads Duberman, 1975 Visher & Visher, 1978, 1979	*acquisition of another's offspring into the family system, i.e., stepchildren, grandchildren, other nonrelated children.
Loss of a spouse (through death, divorce, etc.) Parkes, 1972 Lopata, 1973, 1979 Bohannan, 1970 Wallerstein & Kelly, 1974, 1975, 1976, 1977 Weiss, 1975 Hetherington & Deur, 1971 Hetherington, Cox, & Cox, 1976 Boss & Whitaker, 1979	*separation of mate from the dyad, therefore dissolution of the marital dyad. Note: In case of divorce, the dyad may continue and function on other levels, such as co-parenting, etc.

Table 1 (continued)

Type of Life-Span Family Boundary Changes	Boundary Stressors Related to Physical and Psychological Members in the System
Loss of parent(s) Sheehy, 1976 Silverstone & Hyman, 1976 Levinson et al., 1978	*separation of child from parent(s) (child may likely be an adult)
Formation of a new dyad: remarriage Bernard, 1956 Messinger, 1976 Westoff, 1977 Whiteside, & Auerbach, 1978 Roosevelt & Lofas, 1976	*acquisition of a new mate *acquisition of a new set of in-laws *realignment with family of orientation and former in-laws, children of former marriage, etc. *incorporating or rejecting former friendships, former spouses etc., former spouse may still be in partnership with a member of the new dyad regarding parenting.
Remaining single Stein, 1976	*realignment with family of orientation *if previously married, realignment with former in-laws *acquisition of friends, intimates, colleagues, etc.

From Pauline G. Boss, Normative family stress: Family boundary changes across the life-span. In H.I. McCubbin & P.G. Boss (Eds.), Special issue on stress and coping, *Family Relations*, October 1980, 445-450, p. 448.

must be attempted to manage the stress and/or the emotions (Lazarus, 1966). This recognition of a stressful event or problem by the co-executives is inevitably related to the C factor in the ABCX model described in the previous chapter—the meaning that event has for the family as a whole and for the individual members. Consequently, the recognition itself becomes an additional source of stress and a stressor demanding clarification and resolution.

Clarifying Boundaries

Boundary ambiguity is an especially insidious stressor since it often blocks the coping process. If the person or partners under stress cannot be clear about who is inside and who is outside the family boundaries, then the coping process cannot begin. For example, if a wife is unclear about whether her "workaholic" husband is in or outside of the family, her perception is ambiguous and her cognitive recognition of the problem cannot be fully formed. Specifically, she cannot know if her loneliness is real. After all, she is really not alone; her husband is right there beside her, at least physically. He may be preoccupied or exhausted with his work. Although not alone, she feels lonely; she feels like a single parent, yet she is not. The ambiguity that is pervasive in her marriage and family blocks her ability to make decisions about the situation and her subsequent recognition that she is indeed alone and that her husband is "absent." At least if her husband were dead, she could begin to acknowledge the loss and eventually accept it and reorganize her family into a clear one-parent system. When a mate is both physically and psychologically absent, this lessens the ambiguity and the coping process can begin. Certainly, many couples choose divorce as a way of clarifying an ambiguous and stressful relationship.

What does this mean for the marital partners? When one partner is clear about the absence or presence of the spouse, he or she knows whether to function as a solo executive or a co-executive. It is then possible to define options and roles. By clarifying the leadership in the family system, resources are made clearly available for coping. One does not wait until a mate can come home to balance the checkbook; both learn to manage money, and either one can perform the task if need be.

To illustrate further, a person in a traditional marriage to a psychologically absent but physically present spouse is less able than a single person to find another emotional partner. The resource of an intimate friend is blocked since this particular way of coping would be viewed as being disloyal to the marriage. In one such marriage, where the husband was emotionally unavailable to his wife, he resented her keeping a journal about her feelings. He saw it as competing with his role as spouse, even though he did not have time to listen to her talk about her feelings. His heavy career demands as a military officer, he said, prevented him from giving her the emotional support she needed. However, once he understood that her journal was a *necessary and creative means of coping with his psychological unavailability*, he was able to see that her coping strategy did not threaten their marriage. He also recognized that she would *prefer* to talk with him about many of the things she wrote in her journal. As a result he made himself more psychologically available to her. Their new way of coping as a marital pair was to meet at the officers' club at least once a week, without the children, for a leisurely dinner. The ambiguity in their co-executive relationship was clarified by their joining in discussions of personal and emotional issues, as well as issues about their children, family finances, and so on. Private meetings between co-executives are a critical way of clarifying marital boundaries when one spouse is required to spend more time in work than home activities, if both spouses have demanding jobs, or if time alone together is difficult to manage.

Clarity in Family Communication

It is a cliché to say that good and frequent communication is essential for coping with marital stress, but it is accurate. Even in premarital relationships, couples should attempt to clarify expectations, sharing their goals, joys, and frustrations. If they can define a problem by seeing the ambiguity in their perceptions, they can resolve it much more easily.

Once a couple realizes that job stress is creating a problem for them, they may come up with a variety of solutions. For example, they could reject the high demands of a particular career, perhaps even changing jobs or rejecting promotions. They may decide to invest more time and emotion in their marriage, so that physical presence and psychological presence are more congruent. Or a spouse may make it known clearly to the co-executive mate what times he/she would prefer to be totally available to the family system and on what days or hours he/she is committed elsewhere. This clarity makes coping possible for both mate and children. They understand the reasons for absence and are clear about when the parent will return. Some couples may even find it necessary to make appointments with each other or to tell each other when is a good time to call if they must be absent. This type of specific communication appears to be a major coping strategy for families of busy couples who are heavily committed to their jobs (see Chapter 6).

Families and mates cope with stress by clarifying who is in the family system, when, and on what basis. *Knowing when and how a family member will be available is a major step toward boundary maintenance.* It does not mean mates and family members need to be together all the time; rather, it means they must be clear about when they will be together and when they will not.

Boundary ambiguity can take many forms in a marriage. Table 2 presents some additional examples of how boundary ambiguity can be a stressor in marriage, and how the ambiguity can be clarified.

IMPLICATIONS FOR COUNSELORS AND THERAPISTS

For many couples, clarifying boundary ambiguity is part of their regular communication process. For some couples, though, the help of a counselor or therapist may be needed. The clinician's role may be to support the couple's effort to fortify the boundaries between the couple and their children, between the marital couple and their own parents

TABLE 2
Examples of Ambiguous and Clarified Boundaries

	Ambiguous	Clarified
Individual level	Wife is submissive and childlike in her dependency even though her husband wants her to be more assertive. One can see that her mother is and always has been that way. It appears that her loyalty to her mother is more powerful than her loyalty to herself. She can't change because she says her mother would disapprove.	Wife realizes that the cost of remaining loyal to her mother's submissiveness is too great and so she changes her own behavior to meet her own needs today. She finds less expensive ways to remain loyal to her mother.
Couple level	When one of the mates gets sick, the other gets the same symptoms.	Husband can get sick or even feel blue without wife panicking that it is her fault.
	When husband gets drunk, the wife is drawn into wailing and nagging about why he didn't get home for dinner "for the one millionth time."	When husband gets drunk, wife walks away and does her own thing. At least she doesn't get into the drunken behavior by providing the other half of the dance which could mean nagging or scolding.
Family level	Father abuses his one child consistently because that child reminds him of his older brother who abused him when he was a child.	Father would deal with the anger at his older brother, learn different ways of expressing anger when stressed. Punish the child when the child does something wrong, but not just for triggering memories of his childhood and not abusively.

or in-laws, between the marital couple and the community, or between the partners themselves.

Based on the assumption that married couples are co-executives of the family, the following may be taken as guidelines for professionals who work with ambiguously bounded families.

1) See the marital pair together, in the same room at the same time. Whether you are a teacher, a nurse, a social worker, a money management counselor, or a family therapist, assume the husband and wife are co-executives. Do nothing to split the two. If they are not co-executives—if one or the other seems to be making all the decisions—stimulate them to work toward

effective teaming. Be respectful of their values; teaming can take place in traditional as well as more egalitarian marital systems.

2) See the couple with all of the children; also see the whole group with the grandparents, one set at a time. Having the three generations together is valuable in gaining information about the perceptions of family boundaries at all three levels. Often family members find that just trying to get everyone together for such family meetings has clarified issues for them.

3) Encourage the husband and wife to be alone at times. You may have to teach them how to do this or support their initiative in creating ways to be alone together. Interference from others, such as children and grandparents or employers, should be blocked.

4) In family sessions, help the family draw boundaries which allow the children access to both parents (Minuchin, 1974). In other words, the children must know that they are part of the system but that they are excluded from the marital executive relationships. In this way, they are free to be children and will not become parentified children.

5) As part of developing and strengthening the marital executive pair, support the mates in their check and balance of each other regarding family boundaries. If one appears to be crossing boundaries (e.g., a child acting as a parent), then the other should be free to challenge or leave. Dealing openly with conflict in a healthy and fair way is more functional in reducing stress in family systems than is weak or unbalanced leadership with no apparent conflict between the partners. A wife, therefore, needs to be free and able to challenge her husband's authority, just as he should be free and able to challenge hers.

6) Help to show the couple that they can be loyal to their parents and children without being reactive to their every wish and need. Point out that the time, energy, and resources spent on children and grandparents will vary over the life span. Couples need help in knowing when to respond and take loved ones in and when to close boundaries.

7) Support each mate in his or her individual psychological development and in developing self-sufficiency in problem-solving and in performing all family roles. A wife should be encouraged to occasionally take over some of her husband's usual family roles, like looking after the family car, while he may plan to spend more time on caring for children.

CONCLUSION

Boundary-related marital problems will continue to be stressful until boundaries can be clarified and both agree on (a) who in the partnership performs what roles and tasks, and (b) how they and other family members perceive the situation. Challenges to the family's capacity for boundary maintenance come not only from outside forces, but also from normal developmental maturation throughout the life cycle. Such challenges can be met by spouses' altering their roles and perceptions of who is in and who is out of the family system.

This area of marital stress is a rich one for research. Recognizing and investigating variability in and structure of boundary maintenance is one promising approach to the question of why some marital partners can cope with everyday stressors in their relationship and others cannot.

3

Sexuality: Developing Togetherness

KAYE L. ZUENGLER and

GERHARD NEUBECK

Thirteen-year-old Joe was at least a head taller than the other kids in his class, and his deepening voice sometimes cracked when he answered a teacher's question in class. He now had pubic hair, and often at night he would have erections and wet dreams that would stain the bedsheets. Joe knew only a little about these changes and exactly what was happening to him. When he asked his parents about it they seemed so embarrassed, almost angry, that he did not learn very much. Besides, he did not like to admit that he did not know. His parents were not sure he was ready to learn about sexual matters, and they did not know what to say to him. Although Joe's questions and his changing body were upsetting to his mother and father, the two rarely discussed the matter themselves. So Joe mainly got information from friends, from school, and a little from TV or magazines. But he also learned his parents' negative attitudes towards sex and internalized them.

Jack and Karen, both 29, had been married for over two years. Karen had been unhappy about their sexual relationship for some time. She seemed unable to have an orgasm. At first, she had hoped that things would get better over time, but both partners felt too shy to suggest trying anything new. Then she began worrying that she wasn't normal and wondered if Jack found sex satisfying with her.
Whenever she worked up the courage to discuss the problem, or even hint at her feelings, Jack would get very tense, and they usually ended up quarreling. In a way, it was easier to put up with her disappointment and not rock the boat of her marriage.

These two all too common situations are examples of how sexuality can cause stress in families. Although sexual changes, like other kinds of changes, require adaptation and adjustment by the family, it is our thesis that the failure to talk openly and frankly about sexuality and sexual feelings is the principal source of sexuality-related stress for families. There is, in many American families, a conspiracy of silence regarding the sexuality of their members. It is the rare family which openly communicates about sexual matters, where, for instance, parents and children can frankly talk about menstruation or masturbation. While public discussion about sex is somewhat more acceptable than it used to be, the intimacy of the family relationships seems to make it more difficult to share information and exchange views on sex.

It is clear to us that the conspiracy of silence and defensiveness about sexuality act as stressors in the lives of many, if not most, American families—for individual family members as well as the family as a whole. This silence and defensiveness are part of the aA factor in the Double ABCX Model; an existing intrafamily strain which heightens the specific sexuality-related change and makes it more difficult to deal with.

In this chapter, we will review how sexuality is dealt with in families through *rules, roles,* and *myths.* We will then discuss the phases of sexual development over the life cycle, as well as the particular stressors each phase brings, and suggest some ways of coping with the specific stressors.

ROOTS OF SEXUALITY: FAMILY RULES,
ROLES, AND MYTHS

"Sexuality" is shorthand for a complex phenomenon. First there are the biological givens; we are male and female. Then there is the sex drive, an innate state that includes hormonal, neurological, and psychological components. And finally there are behaviors which spring from this drive. The behaviors in turn are governed by family and cultural beliefs which determine different psychological meanings for different people about sexual acts. In sum, it can be said that our brain is the most important sexual organ.

Many of our behaviors and our attitudes toward sexuality are rooted in our family of origin—in the rules, roles, and myths our families have established. For example, we learn attitudes of guilt or disapproval towards premarital sex, and we have expectations about what sexual behaviors (e.g., aggressive, passive) are masculine or feminine.

> *The Johnston family is under stress. Mother and father have been very open about their sexuality—openly displaying sexual contact, wandering nude in the home, and encouraging sex-related discussion in the home. However, they have very strict but inconsistently applied rules about sexuality for their two adolescents (Jan, age 16, and John, age 18). Jan is punished severely for being in the nude and criticized for indicating interest in boys; John is encouraged to brag about his sexual exploits with girls and is allowed to emulate his father's behavior—almost anytime. The arguments between mother and Jan are explosive!*

A family might have rules (i.e., expectations members are expected to fulfill and follow) to define sexual behavior. For example, there may be a restriction against running around the house in underclothes or a rule about not having opposite-sex friends of adolescent children spend the night. It is important to realize that not all rules are overtly stated; while parents may openly declare a certain "racy" television program off limits to children, there may be an unspoken understanding that, say, homosexuality is "never" to be discussed. Both kinds of rules operate in families, and both are effective ways of passing on attitudes about sexuality.

Defining sex roles (i.e., behaviors, attitudes, feelings expected of males or females) is another way to teach sexual behavior and attitudes. It is assumed in many families that boys do such tasks as taking out the garbage, while girls help in the kitchen. Behavior and expectations are governed according to sex in many aspects of our lives, and children learn very early what is "masculine" behavior and what is "feminine" behavior. For example, many men learn that their identity as a male depends on their readiness to "score" (have sexual intercourse with the opposite sex) whenever and wherever possible. Many women learn that they should be passive and always ready to submit to the sexual advances of men. Although the subject of how sex roles are learned and how these roles affect our future choices is a very important one, we can only touch upon this topic. The important point for our purposes is that once learned, sex-role expectations, or vestiges of them, remain with people all their lives.

Third, a family has certain myths (i.e., inaccurate or distorted accounts of family behavior) about sexual behavior that influence what children expect of themselves and others "No one in our family ever masturbated." "All women in our family were virgins when they married." These false beliefs can play on a child's feelings of family pride and cohesion and can generate strong feelings of guilt if a child believes that his or her behavior has violated these codes. These myths may, of course, be very far from the truth.

These rules, roles, and myths are part of very complex processes of family functioning and serve the purpose of helping families to teach, manage, and control sexuality in the family. What one family defines as acceptable sexual behavior may be quite different from the definition in another family, although families of the same socioeconomic background or racial-ethnic group may share certain expectations and values. When rules, roles, or myths are violated, contradicted, or questioned, family stress is the likely outcome. For example, the definition of a sexual event may differ from member to member. A family rule may seem to be violated when a teenage girl is upset by what she experiences as sexual advances from her father. In the role of father, he may only be showing affection for his "little girl." When different family members either misinterpret or do not openly share their interpretation, misunderstandings can arise which in turn produce stress.

SEXUALITY OVER THE LIFE CYCLE: SOURCES OF STRESS

Each stage of sexual development of each family member brings its own stressful changes, to which the individual and the family must adapt. In this section we will outline the biological changes at each stage, identify the stressors for the family, and, in some cases, note specific coping strategies of families who have managed these stressors.

Prepuberty Sexual Development

Children have a natural curiosity about their bodies. By preschool age most of them can identify the parts of the body and relate to the concepts of "boy" versus "girl." Toilet training, a task to be mastered, has usually taught the child about privacy and bodily functions. The words used to give messages to the child about bodily functions are important ones. Sometimes the words (e.g., "cover up," "bloody mess") convey to the child that the bodily functions are bad, shameful or disgusting. For some children the internalization of those messages results in development of a negative body image and low self-esteem (i.e., if my body is bad, I am bad).

One developmental task in childhood is to integrate a gender identity with other social identities (Nass, Libby, & Fisher, 1981; Newman & Newman, 1979). In play, the child may imitate parental behaviors as a way to discover male-female differences. Sex play, like doctor-nurse roles, is common in childhood. Through play, the child is defining what it means for him/her to be a male or a female. Comparisons of body size, penis or absence of penis, and breast size are made. There is concern about male-female differences in the family, (e.g., who sleeps with whom, how babies are made and born, interest in dressing and bathing). Some children might have feelings about being a girl and not a boy, or vice versa. Some may desire breasts and pubic hair like mom or a penis and hair on the chest and face like dad. Some children will have questions about their own rate of development, the size of the penis, when whiskers can be seen on the face. Some children may experience doubts that they *will* mature and fear of the expectations associated with sexual maturity.

Prepubertal children are responsive to what parents do. They notice hugging, kissing, and stroking. Oftentimes they seek physical comforts from the parents and at the same time try to define themselves as "grown-ups," moving away from the parents. Viewing parents as they kiss, stroke, hug, and hold hands may take on new meaning for the child, both in relation to his/her parents and in fantasized relationships with peers. The child is developing an impression of the self as an intimate, physically loving, sexual human being, thus parental and peer response to him/her is important in consolidating the many changes into a perception of the self.

Many children grow up in families where they are able to observe a mother who is pregnant. They wonder whether the baby eats, sleeps, urinates, and how it will "get out." This is a unique opportunity for parents to educate their children about sex and reproduction, and parents can help cope with the child's confusion by talking with him or her, and by not thinking that the child is too young to understand. In addition, they can guide their offspring toward responsible sex as the issues of sexuality are openly discussed. Particularly important are the messages about values and myths surrounding sexuality (Woods, 1979).

By school age a child develops a sense and a need for modesty and privacy. Playing in sex-segregated groups is more common at this stage of development. There is sensitivity to physical body changes, breast size, penis size, appearance of facial, pubic and underarm hair, and masturbation. Masturbation may take on a new meaning at this phase of development. The child may discover that physical manipulation of the genitals feels good and that the physical touching of the body enhances the appreciation of the physical changes that are occurring. Same-sex chums are important for social support, affirmation of a physical identity, and recognition that one is not "alone" in experiencing physical, psychological, and emotional changes.

By preteen years the individual may feel anxious about the myriad of physical and emotional changes that are taking place. Ambivalent feelings may surface as the child moves away from the dependency and security of the earlier phases of development to the uncertainty, change, and greater expectation associated with adolescence. Changes such as nocturnal emissions, menstruation, feelings associated with masturbation, may evoke feelings of fear, joy, embarrassment, or relief. Most preteens vacillate from feeling alone with all of the changes to a need for peer-comparisons as they accept their new identities.

Parents may become more cautious in relating with their children because of memories of their adolescence and experiences during the heightened sexual development. They may alter their responses to their maturing offspring. Where parents once cuddled, held, kissed, and stroked their children, they may become less physically affectionate with the preteen. Parents may fear homosexuality and respond with less touching of the same-sex child. They may view the impulsivity and emotions of the preteen as frightening. All of this may look frightening to the preteen as well. Communication may become more restrained, less open. The offspring may turn to peers as confidants; this may appear as estrangement to the parents.

To cope with these changes, preteens and their parents need to talk about sexuality and the responsibilities of being sexual individuals.

Sometimes this is best done where outsiders, such as teachers, counselors, or nurses are present, since they are less emotionally involved with the teens than the parents. However, it may be that the bond between parent and preteen can be strengthened where sex is openly discussed in a sensitive, factual, respectful way. In addition, cliques, clubs and "pajama" parties provide outlets for sharing where sex talk occurs among trusted peers. The important component is that the preteen has someone to trust with the intimacies of adolescent development.

Puberty and Growing Up

Puberty produces one of the most dramatic sexual changes in the individual's life: the growth of pubic hair, development of breasts, the menarche, erectile ability and nocturnal emissions, and the discovery of arousal through manipulation of the clitoris and/or vagina or the penis. These changes spell stress for the adolescents and often for the family as well, as our first case example in this chapter showed.

While some boys and girls have been prepared for these developments through some informal education by parents and occasionally more formal instruction at school, or by peers who often provide erroneous information, most kids are taken by surprise. Their bodies and organs perplex them. This stress may be temporary but it will not cease until the adolescents have found a way to deal with their anxieties, search for explanations, and develop a new image associated with their new body and feelings.

Parents, too, are often distressed at this stage. In some families the children are becoming sexually attractive when the parents are feeling less attractive, and this can create tension. Family sexual rules or roles may be the area where the adolescent rebels most strongly against his or her parents.

Since body changes lead to behavioral changes, and ultimately to social behaviors such as dating and its concomitant sexual exchanges, the adolescent may need a new repertoire of behaviors (e.g., asking for a date), attitudes and feelings (e.g., being in love), which are learned mostly by trial and error, and which may produce additional strains and stresses (e.g., shyness, ambivalence). This learning is handicapped by the adolescent's lack of a sexual vocabulary and language; just how to talk to one's friends or lovers about sex is threatening and "risky" and, therefore, stress-producing.

These struggles take place in a permissive society which perpetually bombards the adolescent with sexual cues (e.g., everybody has sex; use of contraceptives is okay), but on the other hand, sends messages (e.g., warnings about pregnancy and sexually transmitted disease) exhorting boys and girls to restrict their sexuality. Masturbation is discouraged; arousal behaviors (at one time called necking and petting) are forbidden. Resolving these dissonances is a constant challenge in the adolescent's life. Usually in our society men are given less dissonance-producing ground rules for their sexual behaviors than women. But for both genders, the stress of finding a mechanism to handle conflicting messages about sexuality is constant.

Interpersonal behaviors engender even more stress. Very little "communication" takes place among adolescents, so a good deal of misreading takes place about the other person's sexual feelings, intentions, know-how, and satisfactions. The adolescent is then caught in an amazingly complex set of circumstances. Living in a society which is ambivalent about sexuality, consumed with curiosity and impulses which he or she cannot yet fully control, having to deal with peer expectations, and the availability of contraceptives and abortion which encourage sexual exploration, adolescents find themselves up against a daily confrontation with their sexuality. This stuggle is unavoidable and constitutes the stress of teenage sexuality.

The Young Adult

Adults, having in the physical sense reached maturity, are faced with the novelty of somehow using their sexual languages. To a degree, the earlier sexual experimentation of adolescence continues on the so-called "singles" scene. Finding a partner with whom sexual relations are a possible consequence provides a challenge and first sexual encounters leading to moderate or full-fledged sexual expression constitute anxiety-laden situations. Every time a new acquaintance looms on the horizon, there is a risk; there is always the possibility that one may be rejected.

Once a relationship has been established on either a casual basis or a long-range or even permanent one, yet another set of stress-provoking events looms at the horizon for lovers. The loss of privacy, undressing and dressing, or the use of the toilet and bath in front of the other, or the use of contraceptives such as the rolling on of a condom in the presence of the partner can be a difficult adjustment. Most couples are able to overcome initial nervousness and settle into routines rather quickly. Some individuals, however, continue to have privacy problems and only gradually learn to cope with the threats which are inherent in being observed and observing.

A second set of issues comes under the heading of performance anxieties: to meet one's own sexual expectations and those of the lover, or to live up to cultural norms which exist or are thought to exist (e.g., frequency of lovemaking). Trying new behaviors (such as assuming different positions in sexual intercourse) may also generate performance anxiety, with each new variation or change presenting an element of stress.

While these are stressors for the individual spouse and/or lover, they obviously affect both partners. We have commented on communication difficulties throughout this chapter and we must emphasize again that these communication difficulties cause a large part of the stress experienced from sexual relations. In our second case example, Jack and Karen felt unable to discuss their private dissatisfaction with their sexual relationship. Not to be able to share anxieties freely, not knowing what the other is feeling or thinking about one's sexual moves or changing patterns, not realizing to what degree these patterns are pleasing or not pleasing and then "sitting" on these concerns generate enormous insecurity. When such pairs consult sex therapists, the first order of business is usually to teach the couple the rudiments of effective communication, beginning often by helping them to use an appropriate vocabulary and then proceeding to get them to speak with each other about sexual matters. This involves not only sharing information, but also sharing feelings. In this way, stress can be alleviated for both partners.

Our sexual attraction to others, as well as the sexual attraction of others to us, is another stress-producing circumstance. Regardless of how we decide to react to sexual attraction, some tension is generated. Also, jealousy comes into prominence and has to be managed.

Marital problems in general create stress, and sexual problems in marriage do the same. Bouts with impotence or a struggle to be orgasmic can create stress for the couple over and above the communication aspects discussed before. Spouses or lovers dealing with what they experience to be a sexual dysfunction usually need professional help; sex therapy has proven to be very effective.

Pregnancy

Pregnancy can be an especially intimate time for a couple—psychologically, physically, emotionally and sexually. Sexuality, though, may take on a different meaning for the couple both during and after pregnancy.

Pregnancy brings physical changes in the size and shape of a woman's body, physical symptoms such as nausea or fatigue, plus changed feelings in both partners about her body. Both partners are slowly getting used to thinking of themselves as parents. These changes require some adaptation if a satisfactory sexual relationship is to be maintained during this period. Some couples feel that they should abstain from coitus altogether, although this is not usually necessary. Masturbation of self and partner brings satisfaction and can reinforce feelings of pleasure, intimacy, love, and closeness. For others, oral sex and altered coital positions bring satisfaction while continuing to respect the physical changes that occur as the woman's body changes.

Coping with the stressors of pregnancy is a couple task. Each trimester requires new coping responses. Many of these responses are a result of the shared experience of the couple. Other people often are in positions to assist the couple with coping and facilitate the shared pregnancy experience. Anticipatory guidance by health care providers, where factual information and suggestions are offered, alleviates fears and reduces the feeling of crisis that some couples experience. Such guidance has been found useful for women in accepting their body-image changes (Weinberg, 1978).

A reflective probing of problems and an ability to talk about their experiences and expectations can reduce stress and anxiety for the couple. Through ventilation of fears, joys, frustration, and clarification of a stressful situation, a couple can offer solutions to problems and lean on each other for support.

In addition to partner support, the pregnant couple can benefit from interaction with their social network. Studies show that social support from others moderates stress (Cobb, 1976) and lessens psychiatric symptoms (Lin, Simeone, Ensel & Kuo, 1979). The social network of health care providers, birth education instructors and coaches, other pregnant couples, family and relatives provides an opportunity for the couple to share their experiences, receive affirmation, and put the pregnancy in perspective with other events in their social world. Childbirth classes are useful in allaying fears about the physical and psychological aspects of labor and childbirth (Newman & Newman, 1979). Couples' support groups that continue after the birth of the baby provide a forum for discussion and give the message that the couple is not alone (Miller & Newman, 1978).

The postpartum time is a special time which requires some additional adjustment. The couple, while getting used to the nonpregnant state, can enhance their sexual communication by using various positions for intercourse and by focusing on mutual pleasure and comfort behaviors other than intercourse.

Both partners are vulnerable to the time-consuming demands of caring for a newborn, but their own emotional and psychological needs demand attention too. Each one needs reassurance that he or she is still loved by the partner. A woman needs to know that her body is still attractive to her partner, that he does not fear the changes in her breasts, vagina, or abdomen. Some women fear that they will not be able to satisfy their partners again. They need reassurance that this is not happening.

Couples need to know that, although lovemaking may be altered during and after pregnancy, they can still enjoy intimacy through sexual relating. Sometimes, by making the necessary adaptations during pregnancy, a couple finds greater and deeper meaning in sexual loving than at any other time in their life together.

Middle Age and Aging

Middle age, like adolescence, is a time of self-doubt and change (Levinson et al., 1978). It is a time when one's own children are becoming teenagers or young adults, or having children of their own, and when one's parents are aging and dying; these visible changes at both ends of the life cycle heighten one's perception of what it means to be growing older. Both men and women may be reflecting on their lives and reexamining their values. Sexual values are also changing. Married couples may feel that sex has become secure but boring; extramarital relationships often begin at this time. Women going through menopause may feel ambivalent about sex. On the one hand, declining estrogen levels may decrease sexual desire for some women. Other women may feel unfeminine when they are no longer able to have children. On the other hand, the freedom from worry about getting pregnant helps some women relax and enjoy sex more. Both men and women worry about how attractive they are.

This can be a shaky emotional time for the intimate couple. Where there are doubts about one's physical appearance, there are generally concomitant doubts about one's desirability and lovability. Where there is a concern about one's ability to perform sexually, there may be either a lack of desire (in women usually) or a need to show that one is still capable in the sexual arena (in men usually). The answer is to change and adapt. A couple needs good communication patterns based on mutual patience and trust, as well as a little courage to be adventurous and playful in a sexual relationship where routine has been the order of the night.

As people reach age 65 or 70, their bodies and energy levels slow down. One of the most frequently occuring sexual problems in older people is a waning sexual desire (Kaplan, 1979). Illness becomes more frequent and may affect both the physical and psychological aspects of sexuality. Men experience occasional erection failures and are often concerned about impotence.

Cleveland (1974) addressed the problem of stress caused by physiological change in the aging male and female. She suggested being less concerned with orgasms and more with intimacy and pleasure. Perhaps as the public begins to accept the legitimacy of sexuality for the aging population, new approaches to sexual relations after age 60 may become more common knowledge.

COPING WITH SEXUALITY: THREE BASIC PRINCIPLES

As we have reviewed the stressors on families associated with each stage of sexual development, we have tried to suggest ways to manage these problems. The most important principles in coping with stressors of sexuality are *communication* among family members, *education* about sexuality, and *getting professional help* when it is needed.

The two examples at the beginning of the chapter presented normal problematic stages in our sexual life cycle—reaching puberty and developing a satisfying sexual relationship. In both cases, the situation was complicated by the family members' inability to talk comfortably with one another about sex, to admit their ignorance, to relax and have a sense of humor about the situation. These reactions might be termed dysfunctional coping methods; the failure to communicate only heightened the stress. Parents and children or sexual partners who can talk about sexual issues are much more likely to cope successfully with inevitable sexual change. Parents should look for opportunities to talk about sex with their children and be sensitive to their confusions and anxieties.

When sexual problems of any kind are defined by our society as shameful, as some indication of deep failure as a male or female, stress is one result. More and valid *information* about sexuality can help couples put the situation into perspective. Attending a sex education class or finding a good book on the subject can be a useful means of coping. Adults should not be ashamed to admit to their children or to their partner that they do not know everything about sexual development.

Finally, it is sometimes easier for couples or families to disentangle themselves from their anxieties and difficulties about sex if they seek *help* from a professional. Quite often the task of the therapist is to help the family talk with one another about sex, to give them the vocabulary and the simple but accurate knowledge they need. The presence of an outsider to mediate the problems may be the best way for some families to resolve their difficulties.

IMPLICATIONS FOR TREATMENT AND PUBLIC POLICY

The professional counselor and sex therapist can play an important part in helping families deal with stressful sexual issues. During especially stressful times, such as pregnancy, counselors, physicians, or other professionals need to inform couples about what they might expect, to help them improve communication skills, and generally to demystify the whole world of sex.

Whether or not to teach sex education in schools is a controversial policy issue in many communities. While the best and most powerful sex education comes from the family, schools often can provide children and adolescents with more accurate information about sex. Sex education can be seen as a preventive stress-reducing measure for children, youth, and adults, helping families understand sexual issues and communicate about them without shame.

CONCLUSION

We have looked at an aspect of family life which, because of its delicate character, holds up the red flag of stress continuously through the life cycle, from the cradle to the cane. Since in our culture we are socialized to feel guilty about our sexuality, or at least feel and face an ambiguity about being sexual, and since we consequently have not been taught to talk about sex, spouse to spouse, parent to child, sibling to sibling, we are indeed vulnerable to stress. Preventive measures such as family or formal sex education need to be adopted, so that we can reassess our attitudes and learn a sexual vocabulary. We need to do more research to understand in detail what stages of the sexual life cycle are most stressful for families and why; we need to know how better sexual communication can be developed in families. Once the sexual atmosphere has been cleared of guilt and an easier verbal interchange has come into being, stress will have been greatly reduced.

CHAPTER

4

Parenthood: Stresses and Coping Strategies

BRENT C. MILLER and
JUDITH A. MYERS-WALLS

When Sarah and Bill James brought their infant daughter home from the hospital, they were thrilled and excited, but both admitted to having problems adjusting to the demands of being new parents. Getting used to a baby and meeting their myriad new responsibilities created a lot of stress for the couple.

Their neighbors, the Cabreras, were facing a different stressor of parenting. Their youngest boy had just graduated from high school and was leaving within days to find a job in another state. Mrs. Cabrera worried that he was too young and that after having three children around she'd never get used to cooking for just herself and her husband again. Mr. Cabrera worried that the house was too big for the couple and wanted to sell it. But they both knew that their release from daily parental responsibilities meant more time for themselves, more money for luxuries, and less worry.

DEFINING THE SCOPE OF PARENTHOOD
AND ITS STRESSORS

Parenthood is a normative life experience in the sense that only an estimated 5-7% of the population of the United States and Canada voluntarily chooses not to have children (Veevers & Figley, 1980). This means that about 95% of those who can have children do. It is important to recognize, however, that parent*hood* is a status or role, whereas parent*ing* is a long-term, intensive task or activity. It seems obvious that most parents probably find parent*hood* (having children) considerably easier than parent*ing* (raising them). While few would disagree that the role of parenthood is normative, there is less consensus about the impact of the tasks of parenting. How difficult is the task of raising children? What are the stressors of parenting?

Evidences of Parenting Stress

Some of the most visible yet least accurate indications of parental stress have appeared in the popular news media. For example, several years ago advice columnist Ann Landers asked parents to write and tell her if they would have children again if they could live their lives over. Seventy percent of the parents who responded reported that they would *not* have children again if they could live life over. Apparently Landers' question touched the raw nerves of frazzled parents who responded in disproportionate numbers.

Based on such highly visible popular sources, the obvious, but erroneous, conclusion is that parenting is highly stressful for a majority of parents—so stressful, in fact, that they wish they had never had children. More accurate data than Landers reported are available, but unfortunately they are less well-known. For example, approximately 90% of a scientific national random sample of 2102 parents (General Mills American Family Report, 1977) would choose parenthood a second time around.

Although the overwhelming majority of parents would choose to have children again, this does not mean that parenting is not stressful. One way of assessing the effects of children on their parents is to compare the stresses and satisfactions reported by parents with those reported by nonparents. In such bald comparisons of those with and without children, childless couples have been found to have higher marital satisfaction (Renee, 1970), a higher frequency of positive couple interaction (Rosenblatt, 1974), and a higher sense of personal well-being (Campbell,

Converse, & Rodgers, 1976). Parents who have children living at home appear to have less satisfying marriages and be under more stress than either young couples who have not yet had children or older parents whose children are no longer living at home (Feldman, 1965; Miller, 1976).

Another indication that parenthood elicits some feelings of stress is that 36% of a nationwide sample of parents in a recent General Mills survey reported that they worry about the job they are doing as parents (General Mills American Family Report, 1977). This worry appears to be translated by some parents into a desire for information, as evidenced by the popularity of the over 200 current book titles for parents (Clarke-Stewart, 1978) and the fact that childrearing was discovered to be the most popular category among the literature titles ordered from the U.S. Government Printing Office in a recent year.

Examples of Specific Parenting Stressors

Specific stressors of parenting can be considered in three major areas—physical, psychological, and financial. The amount of stress that parents experience in these areas varies, of course, and for each parent the mix and overlap of these parenting concerns change over time, as we will discuss in the next section.

Physical Stressors. Even before a child is born, the parents, especially the expectant mother, are likely to experience some physical stress. Approximately half of pregnant women experience nausea and morning sickness during the first trimester. Of course some pregnancies cause prolonged sickness and physical complications, particularly later in pregnancy. Most couples experience an interruption or decline in their sexual relationship during late pregnancy and during the postpartum period (Masters & Johnson, 1966). Young parents are also particularly likely to physically rearrange their living quarters or move into larger accommodations as children are born. Moving might alleviate crowdedness, but there are also stressors associated with changing residences and moving belongings.

Physical stressors are probably most pronounced during the years when children are young. Infants particularly require physical exertion, often to the point of being stressful. LaRossa and LaRossa (1981) found that the management of time was a major issue for new parents. Similarly, Sollie and Miller (1980) found that, when new parents were asked to write about the positive and negative experiences of having the first infant, the most frequent negative response centered around physical demands. The physical demands new parents cited most often had to do with direct caregiving activities including feeding, diaper changing, bathing, comforting/soothing, laundering, etc. During the transition to parenthood it is not unusual for new parents, especially mothers, to report being worn out, fatigued, or exhausted. Physical stressors continue throughout the parenting experience—but perhaps less intensively than when children are very young and dependent.

Psychological Stressors. Although less tangible than physical stressors, the psychological stressors of parenting are real and prevalent. Physical stressors might decline as children grow older and more independent, but psychological stressors probably increase until launching. Simply put, parents worry about their children. They worry about where they are, if they are safe, and how they are doing as compared to their peers. Parents also worry about how they themselves are doing as parents.

Part of the emotional stress of parenting arises out of a concern for the safety and well-being of the child(ren). Parents feel anxiety when their child is in physical or social danger. Parents often fear that their children will be hurt or treated unfairly by others. Likewise, parents grieve over the choices and actions of their children which are likely to result in unhappiness and pain.

Another aspect of the psychological stress of parenting is the child's reflection upon the parent. Just as parents take pride in their children's growth and accomplishments, they are emotionally hurt, sometimes devastated, by their children's slowness, failures, and misdoings. In North America, parents are viewed as being highly responsible for their children and what they become (LeMasters, 1970). Parenting is particularly difficult and stressful when children do not "measure up" to parental or community expectations. In the most extreme cases of psychological/emotional stress, parents anguish over severing or renouncing their relationship with a child rather than continuing to be identified with their unacceptable or socially disapproved behaviors.

Financial Stressors. At one time having many children was an economic asset; they could provide inexpensive labor for the family work that needed to be done. Even today in some countries children are desired for their economic value, in terms of both providing labor and caring for aged parents (Bulatto, 1975; Mueller, 1972; Nag, 1972).

By contrast, it is a cold hard fact that raising children in contemporary Western societies is expensive. In the United States in 1980 the direct cost of raising a child to age 18 was estimated to be about $85,000 for the average family (Espenshade, 1980). The direct maintenance costs include out-of-pocket expenses for childbirth, food, clothing, housing, and education. Of course, this estimated cost can be reduced in various ways, but it can also be considerably more expensive if indirect costs are included. The indirect costs most often added to direct maintenance costs are referred to as opportunity costs, or opportunities foregone by women who stay out of the labor market to have and raise children. If both direct and opportunity costs (potential income) are taken into account, estimates of the average costs of raising and sending a child through four years of college are between $100,000 and $140,000, based on the median family income in the United States (Espenshade, 1980). Although specific dollar figures rapidly become outdated by inflation, a general rule of thumb is that the average direct costs of raising a child from birth to age 18 are about three or four times the family's annual income.

By any method of calculation, the financial costs of raising children are considerable, but the financial stress of parenting encompasses more than just coming up with the necessary money. Financial strains also result from disagreements between parents, as well as between parents and children, about how money should be spent. It is clear, for example, that financial needs and resources are most discrepant during the child-bearing years, but economic disagreement, dissatisfaction, and worries appear to peak with school-aged and adolescent children (Aldous & Hill, 1969). If the assumption is accepted that most families have less money than they would like to have, it follows logically that some stress is likely to occur in deciding how to distribute too little money among too many competing alternatives.

Summary of Specific Parenting Stressors

A variety of stressors associated with parenthood and parenting have been noted above, but there are other problems and difficulties that do not fit nicely into physical, psychological, or financial pigeonholes. In studies about the values and costs of children, several other potentially stressful aspects of parenting have been identified. Perhaps the most commonly mentioned one is the loss of personal freedom parenting entails (Burnside, 1978; Hoffman & Manis, 1979). Another perceived disadvantage of children is less time and companionship in marriage (Barnett & MacDonald, 1976; Fawcett, 1972). Having difficult children or children with serious handicaps appears to increase strains on marriage (Drotar, Baskiewicz, Irvin, Kennell, & Klaus, 1967) and result in a higher likelihood of divorce (Tew, Laurence, Payne, & Rawnsley, 1977). It should be emphasized that these are the potential and probable stressors of parenting; they are not inevitable.

TRANSITIONS IN AND OUT OF PARENTHOOD

One method of acquiring a more detailed assessment of parenting stress is to concentrate on the experiences of parents at two points in time—at the onset and the ending of the period of the most intensive parenting responsibilities. Our two case study families, the Jameses and the Cabreras, illustrate these two transitions. Logically, it makes sense to look at the patterns of stressors and strains along with satisfactions at the time when children first enter the family and when they leave home. These are the two most salient critical role transition points as far as parenting is concerned. There have been many studies about crises, adjustments, and stresses during the transition to parenthood, and there have recently been some very interesting studies of marital and personal qualities as parenting activities are relinquished.

The Transition to Parenthood

For the large majority of adults, one of the sharpest changes in life is having the first child. In fact, Rossi (1968) has stated that the major transition from adolescence to adulthood, especially for a woman, is not marriage but parenthood. The roles and tasks of parenting are acquired abruptly. As soon as the first infant is born, and certainly by the time parents go home from the hospital, they have parental roles—there are social expectations about what they should do. By comparison, later normative changes during the parental career occur much more gradually, as children become toddlers, school children, teenagers, and then young adults on their own. There is, then, a point in time when parental roles are abruptly acquired, but there is also a more gradual transition into the many skills and routines of parenting. Although the transition to parenthood is considered a "critical role transition point," it is also a phase or span of time (Aldous, 1978).

Based on Hill's (1949) conceptualization that accession, or adding a family member, would constitute a "crisis," i.e., a sharp change for which old patterns were inadequate, LeMasters (1957) conducted the first study of parenthood as a crisis. He found, as did Dyer (1963), that a majority of middle-class parents experienced "extensive or severe" crisis as defined above. Both of these studies can be faulted for small unrepresentative samples and the LeMasters study for probable experimenter effects (Rosenthal, 1966) because he helped the couples decide how much crisis they had experienced.

The term "crisis" as an appropriate designation has also been criticized because the transition to parenthood is generally considered to be a normal event. Because of this, Rapaport (1963) suggested the term "normal crisis," and Rossi (1968) advocated dropping references to crisis altogether: "There is an uncomfortable incongruity in speaking of any crisis as normal. If the transition is achieved and if a successful reintegration . . . occurs, then crisis is a misnomer" (p. 28). After Rossi's classic essay, the term crisis has been used less to refer to the transition to parenthood.

Hobbs (1965, 1968) and Jacoby (1969) reported much lower levels of crisis experienced by new parents than either LeMasters or Dyer had found. More recent studies (Hobbs & Cole, 1976; Hobbs & Wimbish, 1977; Miller & Sollie, 1980; Russell, 1974) have arrived at similar conclusions. Part of the discrepancy between the earlier and later studies seems to be due to focusing on different aspects of the transition; recent studies have focused more on reactions to changes (feelings and attitudes) rather than on the changes (behavior patterns) themselves. The Hobbs checklist, for example, asks questions about how "bothered" parents were about various problems of new parents; only small amounts of "crisis" have been found when parents are questioned in this way. Some researchers have suggested that the behavioral changes accompanying new parenthood are typically extensive, but most new parents are only slightly or mildly bothered by these changes, and a large number report gratifications arising from first parenthood as well (Russell, 1974; Steffensmeier, 1978). Myers-Walls (1979) found that the amount of life-style change was negatively related to the parents' ability to accept the changes, but parents who felt positive about the changes in their lives as a result of the baby also reported experiencing more parenting satisfactions and joys.

Social desirability has also been a methodological problem in studying changes or reactions during the transition to parenthood. When the researcher connects children and problems by asking the new parents to tell how bothered they are, or how much things have changed, a nagging doubt arises about how truthful parents will be. Because of the strongly pronatalist and romantic view of children in American society

(LeMasters, 1970), it is difficult for new parents to objectively answer questions about how children have changed their lives. Consequently, there is some question about the validity of their self-reports.

Another general criticism of most transition to parenthood research is that it has usually been conducted after the fact. When changes and their accompanying stresses are to be studied, inferential validity is stronger if subjects are assessed both before and after the child. With before and after measures, changes do not have to be recalled or estimated by the new parents—they can be calculated by the researcher directly. In one longitudinal study of this kind, Feldman (1971) found declining marital satisfaction between five months of pregnancy and five months postpartum, especially among couples who had the most companionate relationships before parenthood. Ryder (1973), who used a different measure of marital satisfaction, did not find significant decreases in husband or wife scores; he did report, however, that new mothers reported more "lovesickness" (a feeling that their husbands were not paying enough attention to them) after their baby had been born.

In a more recent longitudinal study, Miller and Sollie (1980) assessed personal well-being, personal stress, and marital stress during pregnancy (time 1) and later when the first baby was one month old (time 2) and eight months old (time 3). Both new mothers and new fathers reported higher scores on personal stress items after they had become parents. Wives' personal stress scores during pregnancy were lower than their husbands' scores on the average, but new mothers ended up with higher personal stress scores than their husbands. Personal well-being scores of new mothers were lower at time 3 than at time 2, and personal well-being for fathers was lower at time 3 than during the pregnancy observation and when the baby was about one month old.

The most interesting sex difference in the changes was evident on the marital stress scale. New mothers reported higher stress in their marriages after the baby had been born than before, and even higher marital stress by the time the baby was about eight months old. New fathers' marital stress scores, by contrast, remained essentially the same across the year of the study. These data coincide with Ryder's (1973) finding that new mothers were more likely than fathers to report that their spouses were not paying enough attention to them.

In summary, parents are clearly affected by the first experience of assuming parental roles. In a classic article about the transition to parenthood, Rossi (1968) pointed out that it is unlike any other role in life. Most of what parents know about parenting is acquired haphazardly through socialization when they were children themselves; there is typically little, if any, formal preparation. It is even more sobering that parental roles are virtually irrevocable. In contrast to work and marital roles, Rossi wrote that "we can have ex-spouses and ex-jobs, but not ex-children." Perhaps the best summary about the amount of stress or "crisis" experienced is that the transition to parenthood for most couples *does* include sharp or decisive changes for which previous patterns of behavior are inadequate, but most parents are only mildly or moderately bothered by these changes. In other words, there is little doubt that having the first child ushers in many significant life changes, usually more so for the mother than the father, but parents do not generally have strong negative reactions to the changes which occur.

Transition to the "Empty Nest"

At the other end of the parenting life cycle there comes a time when day-to-day parenting responsibilities, which may have dominated or been a major organizing feature of the parents' lives, are diminished or relinquished. The concept of postparenthood is a misnomer because the status or role of parent is never given up—once a parent, always a parent. We prefer the term "launching" to refer to the period of time when maturing adolescents leave their families of orientation; this period begins when the first child departs and ends when the last leaves home. The terms "empty nest" and "postparental years" are used to describe the time which begins with the last child's departure and ends with the retirement or death of one or both spouses. The transition or bridging period, spanning the end of launching and the beginning of the empty nest, is especially salient here because this is when parenting stress, if it has been present, should begin to be alleviated.

With the emergence of empty nest marriages in the present century,* folk wisdom has it that this time is difficult for parents, especially for mothers because they typically invest more of themselves in parenting than fathers do. However, research findings about changes in personal feelings and marital relations during launching and postparenthood

---

*An extended couple relationship after children are launched is, historically, a recent phenomenon. In the previous century the last child's leaving home and one spouse's dying approximately coincided, ending both marital and parental careers simultaneously (Glick, 1955). Two centuries ago, the typical pattern was widowed parenthood; in the average family one spouse's death ended the marital career 10 years before the last child left home (Wells, 1973). Today, in the typical North American family the empty nest stage is the longest of the family life cycle, averaging 18 to 20 years (Aldous, 1978; Duvall, 1977).

have been limited and inconsistent. One early study suggested that marital relations during postparenthood were less satisfying to wives than the previous years of marriage had been (Blood & Wolfe, 1960). A recent study of postparenthood reported that most fathers have neutral (35%) or positive (42%) feelings about their last child's leaving home, but 22% of fathers felt some degree of unhappiness (Lewis, Freneau, & Roberts, 1979). Compared with the neutral and positive fathers, those who reported unhappiness were more likely to have fewer children and less satisfying marriages, suggesting that they might have the most to lose with their children's departure.

Other studies have suggested that more difficulties are experienced during the years when children are being launched and that personal and marital feelings become more positive when children are gone (Campbell, Converse, & Rodgers, 1976; Deutscher, 1964; Glenn, 1975; Rollins & Cannon, 1974; Rollins & Feldman, 1970). In any case, the most salient issue is how parents and marriage change *during* the transition from launching to the empty nest; none of the studies to date has actually measured the *changes* over time implied by this research problem.

Most recent evidence from cross-sectional comparisons (comparing couples who have launched children with similarly aged couples whose children are still home) suggests that there are fewer stressors after children are gone. The phenomenon of greater well-being among parents whose children are no longer living at home prompted one researcher to quip, "The nest might be empty, but it's sure comfortable" (Campbell, 1976, p. 117).

STRESS AND PARENTING ACROSS THE LIFE CYCLE

The studies of the establishment and launching stages of parenthood indicate that, indeed, the role is associated with some stress, although the amount of stress is not insurmountable nor unduly severe, and it is tempered with satisfactions. There is still much understanding to be gained, however, from an analysis of the specific stressors which occur during the parenting life cycle. Understanding the stressors during various phases of development is a crucial first step toward learning to cope with these stressors and toward achieving positive growth in the parenting role.

Each time the child enters a new stage (e.g., becomes verbal, starts school, reaches puberty), the parents must learn new role behavior.

Likewise, as parents themselves enter new developmental stages, parenting issues change. At times, the nature of the parents' and children's developmental stages will conflict. Whenever change occurs, there will be a period of stress as parents and children adjust.

Table 1 outlines some of the major issues for children, adults, couples, and parenting at several stages in the parenting life cycle. The life cycle stages are based on the age of the child, although it is recognized that there are difficulties with such a breakdown. One difficulty arises when there are several children of different ages. The issues listed are not mutually exclusive, however, and families may be dealing with issues at several stages simultaneously. A more important concern with this type of chart is that it assumes the parents are married and bearing children in their twenties. The stressors single parents (see Chapter 8), teenage parents, and individuals or couples who postpone parenthood until their thirties are certainly significantly different. Another shortcoming is that the focus of some sections of the table—especially those dealing with the couple relationship—is decidedly negative and problematic. This reflects the tendency of the research literature to deal with problems and conflicts rather than satisfactions and gratifications.

Finally, the reader should keep in mind that any attempt to categorize the experiences of families will be simply that—an attempt. Each individual will have a unique experience during the parenting life cycle. The chart is meant as a generalization of issues which may alert students of the family to frequent difficulties and concerns at specific times. All of these reservations should be kept in mind when using the table as a tool to understand families during the childrearing years.

Although Table 1 presents numerous developments and relationships which merit discussion in more detail, space does not allow for extensive elaboration here.* A further description of three selected issues, i.e. traditionalization of sex roles, maternal employment, and the use of time and energy, however, should help to provide a better understanding of the relationship between stress and parenting across the parenting life cycle.

Traditionalization of Sex Roles

A number of studies have shown that the division of labor within couples follows a more traditional sex-role pattern following the birth

---

*For a more complete discussion of these stages, see Rapoport, Rapoport, and Strelitz (1977) or Aldous (1978).

TABLE 1. Issues for Children, Adults, Couples and Parenting Across the Life Cycle

	TRANSITION INTO PARENTHOOD	PRESCHOOL CHILDREN	SCHOOL-AGE CHILDREN	ADOLESCENTS	LAUNCHING STAGE
ISSUES IN CHILD DEVELOPMENT	Total dependence Vulnerability Total care, maintenance Attachment	Separation/Autonomy Drive for Individuation Aggression Gender Identity Verbal Expression and understanding	Increased Impact of Other Influences Development of Moral Judgments Achievement (Academic, Athletic, Artistic, etc.) Consolidation of Gender Identity Development of Positive Self-Concept	Socialization to Outside Adult World Control of Sexual Impulses Control of Aggressive Impulses Maintenance of Positive Self-Concept Independent Identity Expression of Values	Establishment of Independent Life Style —Financial —Geographical —Emotional —Occupational
ISSUES IN ADULT DEVELOPMENT	Concerned with Making Satisfying Life Investments Preoccupied with being Productive and Performing Well High Financial Stress High Demand on Time and Energy Resources Fathers: —Crucial Stage of Career —May Have Growing Dissatisfaction with "Rat Race" —May Desire to Participate in Childrearing Mothers: —At Risk for Depression, Suicide, Marital Violence, Child Abuse —Fulltime Homemaker at Risk for Social Isolation, Boredom —Employed Mothers at Risk for Overcommitment of Resources			Established Economically Peak or Early Decline of Earning Power Generally Good Health Preoccupied with the Yield from Life Investments/Taking Inventory Beginning of Biological Decline "Middle Generation" Fathers: Slow Down of "Rat Race" Mothers: Fulltime Homemakers—Reassessment of Future	
ISSUES FOR COUPLES	Adjustment to a triad Sharing Love with Another Finding Time to Be Together Traditionalization of Sex Roles	At Risk for End of Marital Honeymoon —Low Ebb of Marital Satisfaction —Poor Communication —Alienation from Each Other's Roles —Disagreements about Finances —High Demand for Decision-Making		At Risk for Reassessment of Marriage and Marital Roles —Disenchantment —"Hollowness" in Relationship —Boredom —Further Alienation from Each Other's Roles	
PARENTING ISSUES	Attachment Type of Child Care Relationship with New Grandparents Division of Parenting Responsibilities Building of Basic Trust in Child	Discipline Establishing Relationships Between —Work and Family —Alternative Child Care and Family —School and Family —Leisure/Recreation and Family Dealing with Childrearing "Experts"	Encouragement of Positive Self-Concept in Child	Setting Limits Allowing Participation in Adult Roles Communication Programming, i.e., Parents vs. Adolescent Determining Activities Values (Religious, Sexual, etc.) Distancing, i.e., Allowing Independence while Communicating Concern Dealing with Conflict between Parent and Adolescent Developmental Stages	

of the first child (Cowan, Cowan, Coie, & Coie, 1978; Entwisle & Doering, 1980). Whereas many of the family tasks and responsibilities may have been shared before the birth of the first child, there tends to be a growing separation and perhaps alienation between male and female roles with the advent of parenthood.

LaRossa and LaRossa (1981) have speculated that this separation may be due to the tendency of women to "embrace" the role of parenthood while men establish "role distance." Other couples may find that the increased time and energy demands during the transition to parenthood simply make it inefficient to try to share all tasks and responsibilities. This need to separate roles usually results in traditionalization, because the couple's background and training will probably have given them greater skills and experience in traditional domains. Of course, the woman's physical involvement in pregnancy, delivery, and postpartum recovery along with a possible commitment to breastfeeding also increase her involvement with parenting roles during the transition into parenthood.

Increased traditionalization is especially stressful for young, middle-class couples who are more likely than others to value an egalitarian marital relationship. Even for those couples who are philosophically comfortable with the role separation, however, the situation can become stressful if the separation results in role alienation and poor communication. The distance between marital partners is likely to increase steadily during the most demanding and active years of parenthood. It is then unlikely that communication patterns will change drastically later, even when the demands on time and energy are reduced as the children grow older and more self-sufficient.

Maternal Employment

Statistics have shown a consistent increase over recent years in the number of mothers who are part of the work force in the United States. No matter what her decision, the issue of employment will affect every American mother and is potentially stressful for her and her family.

Women who are employed during their childbearing and childrearing years are at risk of overcommitting their time and energy resources. Because of the tendency for traditionalization of sex roles among parents, an employed mother often finds herself responsible for two fulltime jobs: one outside the home and one inside. On the other hand, women who are fulltime homemakers during the active parenting years have been found to be at risk for stresses related to the monotony, fragmentation of tasks, and pressures for speed in performance associated with fulltime housework (Oakley, 1974a, 1974b; Rapaport, Rapaport & Strelitz 1977). In addition, fulltime homemakers are faced with making a decision about the placement of their energies and emotional commitments when the children leave home. Finally, employed mothers must deal with the criticism from those who believe mothers should be home with their children, while homemakers are criticized for doing unimportant work or for not living up to their full potential as women.

Use of Time and Energy

Some researchers have found that the greatest concern for new parents is the use of time (LaRossa & LaRossa, 1981). Others have found that those who are able to deal effectively with the time and energy demand of multiple roles tend to adjust to parenthood most easily (Myers-Walls, 1979). The allocation of the limited resources of time and energy is a source of stress for virtually all parents, especially during the early and middle phases of parenting.

Parenting responsiblities are usually added to a person's repertoire during the time of career establishment. This means that the time pressures of caring for a totally dependent infant occur at the same time that one or both parents are investing large amounts of time and energy in learning a relatively new job and earning recognition and promotions in their work. Although the period of total infant dependence is not long, the child's growing independence does not provide significantly greater freedom for the parents for several years, usually after the period of most difficult career adjustment has taken place. The bottom line, then, is the widespread experience of a period of overwhelming time and energy demands for most families with young children.

HOW PARENTS COPE WITH THE STRESSES OF PARENTING

Not all parents find adaptive methods for coping with parenting stresses. One of the most tragic and severe indicators is the level of child abuse and neglect. It has been estimated that over one million children annually are abused by their parents and that between 2,000 and 5,000 die because of parental maltreatment. Several studies have found stress—both parenting stress and stress resulting from other unrelated sources—to be a precipitating factor in child abuse (Fried & Holt, 1980;

Helfer & Kempe, 1976; Kempe & Helfer, 1974; Young, 1964). Further evidence that some parents have difficulty coping with parenting stress is found in rates of child abandonment and observations of indifference in parent-child interactions.

Functional Methods of Coping

Just as little is known about the relationship between stress and parenting, there is also little evidence about which coping strategies are most effective in dealing with that stress. This is a growing area of interest, however, and the information available is increasing rapidly. Current evidence suggests that there are perhaps three primary functional coping techniques used by parents: 1) reliance on support systems and natural helping networks; 2) application of methods for balancing multiple role responsibilities; and 3) the seeking of assistance from professionals and from media sources.

Social Support. Recent work in the area of human services and stress has increasingly studied the operation of naturally occurring helping networks. The terminology used to refer to such networks ranges from informal support systems (Wingspread Report, 1978) to family social networks (Unger & Powell, 1980) to natural neighbors or natural helping networks (Collins & Pancoast, 1976). "The central concept linking all of these terms is the image of lay people helping family, friends, and neighbors in times of need with no expectation of direct compensation" (Myers-Walls & Coward, in press, p. 2).

Indicators of the effectiveness of support systems in helping parents deal with stress are varied. Colletta (1981) states:

> Our research has, in general, reported that being embedded in an active support system is positively related to maternal mental health and negatively related to the frequency of restrictive, demanding, and rejecting interactions with children (p. 1).

She goes on to cite additional studies (Albrecht, 1954; Cannon-Bonvente & Kahn, 1979; Hill, 1970; Reiss, 1962) which uphold the contention that "the extended family is an important resource with aid commonly being in the form of help during illness, financial assistance, childcare or gift giving" (p. 1). This finding is in contrast to Bronfenbrenner's (1974) statements about the contemporary fragmentation and alienation of modern families. In her study of young mothers, Colletta (1981) found that those with high levels of support were more affectionate, closer, and more positive with their children, while those with low levels of support were more hostile, indifferent, and rejecting of their children.

Relating social support to parenting stress, some authors have found that the support did not have a direct effect on parenting behaviors, but did serve to mediate the effects of stress and depression (Longfellow, Zelkowitz, Saunders, & Belle, 1979). Other authors have found that social support is helpful in both areas (Crnic, Greenberg, Ragozin, & Robinson, 1980), and that social support may be an important influence on mother-child relationships in and of itself, not simply a moderating variable acting on stress (Crnic, Greenberg, Ragozin, Robinson, & Basham, 1981).

Not only is support from friends, neighbors, and extended family important, but it appears that a crucial relationship for mothers is with fathers. Zur-Szpiro & Longfellow (1981) found that mothers who described their partners in more positive terms reported less stress in those relationships, felt less depressed, and felt less stressed about their parenting situation. Myers-Walls (unpublished research finding) found that new mothers who expected their husbands to help more with their new babies subsequently adjusted to parenthood more easily than those who did not expect much help.

Thus far the research has shown that social support is an important means for helping parents cope positively with the stresses of parenting. There remain numerous unanswered questions, however. For example, does social support have a direct influence on parenting skills and behavior, or is its most important contribution in coping with stress? Different people in an individual's environment appear to make varying contributions with their support. Which relationships are most important for alleviating parenting stress? How does social support serve to mediate stress? These and other questions should be answered before attempting to develop interventions aimed at reducing stress through increasing social support.

Balancing Roles. Another set of coping techniques has received only limited attention in the literature, although it deals with a stressor commonly mentioned by parents, i.e., having too many responsibilities and too little time and energy to fulfill them. The issue is becoming even more crucial as growing numbers of mothers join the work force. Paloma (1972) looked at working mothers to see if she could identify effective coping strategies for dealing with stress. She first identified those mothers who were coping well and those who were not. By comparing the behaviors of the two groups she was able to identify four techniques which are apparently effective in balancing work and parenthood.

The first of Paloma's (1972) four coping strategies is the ability to deal with guilt and to hold a positive definition of the situation. The second strategy involves the establishment of a salient role. Those mothers who could clearly say which role came first, especially if it was parenthood, coped better with the multiple responsibilities. Compartmentalizing the roles, i.e., concentrating on one set of responsibilities at a time, is the third strategy, while the fourth is a willingness to compromise standards in one or both roles.

Myers-Walls (1979) measured the use of these strategies among new mothers attempting to balance parenthood with work and/or a social life. She found that those parents who made use of these four techniques had an easier transition to parenthood. She also found that the use of the four strategies was *not* successful in the balancing of parenthood with housekeeping responsibilities of the marital role, however.

THE ROLE OF THE PROFESSIONAL IN HELPING PARENTS COPE WITH STRESS

We are living in a time that L. J. Stone has dubbed "the age of self-conscious parenthood" (as cited in Church, 1976, p. 14). Today's parents have moved away from the belief that "Father knows best" or "Mother knows best" and toward the idea that "the experts know best." This is reflected in the popularity of childrearing literature cited earlier. Is this dependence on professionals or "experts" increasing or decreasing the amount of parenting stress experienced by today's mothers and fathers?

There are mixed reports on the effectiveness of intervention by professionals in helping parents deal with stress. This diversity is accounted for partially by the variety of types and styles of intervention they provide. Some of these types are reviewed in more detail below.

Parent Education Classes

One very positive type of intervention has been the childbirth education movement. A number of studies have shown that expectant parents who participate in prepared childbirth classes feel more positive about the birth experience and about the baby and generally cope better during labor and delivery (Dalzell, 1965; Doering & Entwisle, 1975; Hungerford, 1972).

Studies of other types of parent education interventions have not been as promising, however. Myers-Walls (1977) found that greater amounts of training in child development, childbearing, or childrearing tended to be associated with lower amounts of self-confidence among new mothers. However, this might mean that the most confident mothers did not take such classes, not that the classes reduced self-confidence. Reviews of other evaluations of parent education classes have shown that several claim to have positively affected knowledge, attitudes, and behavior of participants (Brim, 1959). A more recent generalization is that parent education:

> can and does have effects on both its participant clientele and upon their children. There is clear, although not abundant, evidence showing that the children of participants are influenced in intellectual, cognitive, mental health, physical health, and affective development (Harman & Brim, 1980).

It appears, then, that parent education classes can be an important source of information for new parents, but that it is possible that they could also increase rather than decrease stress levels by raising expectations or standards. Of course, most evaluation studies have not looked specifically at stress levels as outcome variables, nor have they often been sensitive to possible deleterious outcomes; this limits the conclusions that can be drawn. For instance, it is unclear whether the higher stress levels and lower self-confidence preceded or were a consequence of parent education experiences in the few studies which included these variables. Similar inconclusiveness was reported by Geboy (1981), who found that parents under stress were not necessarily receiving the help they needed from the available child-care literature, in spite of its popularity; the amount of literature read by parents was neither positively nor negatively associated with how much the parent worried about parenting issues.

Parent Support Groups

Wandersman (1981) reported on several programs designed to provide support to new parents. There were, however, many obstacles to a summary of the results. One such obstacle was the tendency of program evaluators to focus on large-scale, relatively stable characteristics as outcome variables, rather than the immediate program goals of building a support network, reducing isolation, and encouraging sharing among peers.

In spite of these methodological weaknesses, there is some indication that participants in support groups tend to report an increase in network affiliations and discussion of child-care (McGuire & Gottlieb, 1979), a recognition of universal feelings among parents (Cronenwett, 1980), and a sense of gain and satisfaction in subjective reports (Wandersman, 1978, 1980). Wandersman (1981) encourages more systematic and goal-oriented investigation of both implementation and evaluation of such programs.

Formal Services Coordinated with Informal Helping Networks

A recent, innovative trend in community programming has been to investigate means of combining formal and informal human service delivery (Myers-Walls & Coward, in press). Much of this programming has been directed towards parents. Research in this area has followed three identifiable lines: 1) the formation and operation of self-help groups (e.g., Parents Anonymous, Parents Without Partners); 2) the provision of human services by community caregivers (e.g., bankers, lawyers, and doctors) above and beyond the scope of their normal job responsibilities; and 3) the extending of emotional and practical assistance by an individual's social intimates—family members and friends (Gottlieb & Schroter, 1978). All of these approaches are potentially useful methods for intervening with stressed parents.

Myers-Walls and Coward (in press) have listed a number of advantages of combining formal and informal service delivery methods, some of which are:

- cost: since informal helpers are not paid and do not use office or secretaries, more people can be served for less money;
- credibility: natural helpers are people from the community who have demonstrated their ability to listen, make referrals, and provide other assistance; therefore, there should by definition be less difficulty with the natural helper being accepted by potential clients;
- reaching isolated populations: because natural helpers normally meet their "clients" in the course of everyday living, they are in an ideal position to reach rural and small-town residents;
- increased independence of clients: the type of assistance provided by informal helpers can be continued indefinitely, unlike that provided by formal agencies, so the weaning of the client from the service delivery system is unnecessary.

Little is available currently in the way of evaluations of programs combining formal and informal delivery formats. What little is available does indicate, however, that the approach is promising and worth further experimentation in this time of diminishing resources. Because the approach is only minimally tied to formal bureaucracies, it appears to be especially well-suited to situations of stress and crisis.

SUMMARY AND CONCLUSIONS

This chapter has focused on the stress of parenting and ways of most effectively coping with this stress. Parenthood is a normative experience, and stress arising from parenting is also normative. It appears, however, that initial parenting experiences are only slightly stressful, on the average. Similarly, personal and marital well-being rises slightly when children leave home. There is, of course, considerable variability around the central tendencies emphasized in this chapter. The stressors of parenting are surely greater, for example, for single parents (see Chapter 8), for parents of handicapped children (see Chapter 2, Volume II), for those who become parents very young, and so on. Like so many family phenomena, the amount of stress experienced in parenting depends on many things, including the family's particular situation, the parents' personal attributes and values, and characteristics of the child(ren).

It should also be acknowledged that parenting stressors are not necessarily harmful or detrimental. Of course, extreme or severe stress may result in violence, abandonment, or abuse; but perhaps the modest stress which appears to be most common is motivating to parents and ultimately helpful to children.

The stressors of parenting are most frequently adapted to through natural or informal means. Family and friends are sought out for advice and direct assistance. However, professionals are increasingly relied on by providing parenting literature, formally organized support groups, and parent education. Parenting, which has always been the pedestrian pursuit of amateurs, is becoming an activity which more people consider thoughtfully and for which they make careful preparations.

5

Parents and Adolescents: Push and Pull of Change

JEANNIE KIDWELL, JUDITH

L. FISCHER, RICHARD M. DUNHAM,

and MARC BARANOWSKI

Mr. and Mrs. Harry Beck spend many hours figuring out what they should do with their 16-year-old daughter, Denise, who is "out with a bunch of wild kids" and sarcastic, if not disrespectful, to them and her younger brother Dennis. In private her parents are afraid that her friends will push Denise to use drugs and to become a "delinquent." They are afraid to be too tough on her for they also feel that Denise needs room to breathe and to stretch her wings; but they also can't stand the way things are going! Down deep, they are angry and demand that Denise abide by the rules; after all, they are parents and children need discipline, and parents are supposed to be in charge. The "experts" Mr. and Mrs. Beck read and listen to are not very consistent; some say give the kids "tough love" and other

The authors wish to acknowledge Groves Workshop participants' stimulation to the discussions which led to this chapter. Gratitude is extended to Walter Schumm for his contribution to the paper.

*say "give them space"; the Becks are confused while they face the
daily battles with Denise and try to settle the fights between Denise
and Dennis. What is happening? Are they an abnormal family to
struggle and feel this way?*

Popular literature and personal anecdotes commonly support the notion that adolescents represent a special source of stress to their parents.
Recently, this idea has been reinforced by the publication of results from
a survey of 30,000 predominantly young middle-class working mothers
in the June 1980 issue of *Ladies Home Journal*. Among the conclusions of
the study were that:

> Women with children under six years old and women with teen-
> agers are under the greatest stress. . . Those with 13- to 17-year
> olds have the roughest time of all . . . (p. 146).

Other research also attests to the stress of parenting teenagers. Research on marital satisfaction, for example, suggests that the marital
relationship suffers most during the phase of the life cycle when the
children are adolescents (Rollins & Feldman, 1970).

Most people assume that the stress resulting from the presence of
teenagers in the home is created by adolescent rebellion, aggressiveness,
drug usage, peer pressure, and other feared behaviors. Pathological
issues, such as anorexia nervosa, schizophrenia, and drug abuse, have
been the focus of most of the academic literature on parent-adolescent
relationships. While behavior problems like drug abuse, anorexia nervosa, or schizophrenia are no doubt serious stressors, it is our belief that
much of the stress experienced by families during the adolescent years
arises out of normative life stage developmental events, experienced to
varying degrees in *all* families in which there is an adolescent.

There are numerous transitions in the development of parenting. The
initial transition to parenthood has received considerable research attention, while the transition to parenting an adolescent or a young adult
has received limited attention. This chapter is, therefore, concerned with
normal life stresses of transitions in parenthood, specifically, parenting
an adolescent. We draw upon systems theory to provide a conceptual
framework which brings into focus specific transitional events during
this stage of the family life cycle and shows how these transitions might
produce stress. Efforts to clarify transitional issues under a comprehensive framework are important in several ways: for understanding functional and dysfunctional ways in which families cope with this stressor;

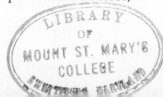

for further development of service delivery and intervention strategies; and for the direction of future research.

The chapter begins with a brief overview of some of the critical developmental changes within the adolescent and discusses some behavioral implications of these changes. The developmental events which are discussed are cognitive development and identity formation. In addition, the parents as individuals undergo developmental changes of their own, and these changes also have implications for family functioning and parenting. Within a systems framework, these transitional events of adolescents and their parents are viewed as potential catalysts for creating stress and producing changes in a family system which has been operating with preadolescent children. Ways in which family systems operate to cope with these stresses are discussed. Throughout the chapter it is recognized that the stresses in adolescence are culturally bound. That is, the stresses of adolescence are not recognized as taking the same form universally but are seen as specific to certain societies. Our discussion centers on Western industrialized societies, such as the United States.

CRITICAL DEVELOPMENTAL CHANGES IN ADOLESCENCE

The aim of this section is to provide a brief overview of some of the critical developmental events occurring during the stage of adolescence. An understanding of these changes and the observable behaviors arising out of them serves as a background for discussing the effects on a family system when one or more of its members are in a critical developmental transition—often referred to as a "developmental crisis." Erikson (1968, p.15), for example, labels adolescence as a period of crisis, and he defines crisis as: "a necessary turning point, a crucial moment when development must move one way or another, marshalling resources of growth, recovery, and further differentiation."

Several important events occur during pubescence which influence the individual to marshall his or her own resources of growth for further differentiation. The most obvious are, of course, the physiological changes. The greater size, growth of body hair, voice changes, and other outward manifestations of growing reproductive capacity all send strong signals to the adolescent, to his or her parents, and to the immediate society, that the young person is becoming an adult. Less obvious, but of considerable importance, are cognitive and identity changes.

Cognitive Changes

Similar to physiological changes, cognitive changes also result in observable manifestations of an individual in transition to adulthood. Piaget's work on cognitive development reveals these developmental changes. As with all development, adolescence is characterized by a progression through an invariant sequence of organized structures of thought and action. These structures of thought and action are constructed by the individual and undergo successive changes through interaction with the social and physical environment. These changes in structure are designated as stages. In all stages there are qualitative changes in modes of thinking (Inhelder & Piaget, 1958).

Piaget emphasizes three interrelated activities which are necessary for an individual's cognitive and social development: reflection, decentering, and the ability to take the roles of others. In adolescence, the individual is undergoing a rather rapid restructuring of thought processes, involving all three of these activities. Reflection means paying attention to one's own thought processes and checking to make certain that one is taking account of the interrelations of several aspects of the problem. The process of trying to communicate one's own reasoning to another person requires reflection because it forces one to decenter—to look at a problem from another person's perspective and not just one's own. Decentering requires one to take the role of another. "Consciousness of one's own reasoning processes arises from the disposition to prove and justify to others what one has asserted: to do the latter one must turn back upon, reflect on, one's own thinking critically, and with the eyes of an outside observer" (Flavell, 1963, p. 279). Communication entails reflection; reflection is built upon decentering and decentering is fostered by having to take the points of view or "roles" of others.

These changing thought processes in adolescence are often referred to as the development of formal operational thought or formal operations (Inhelder & Piaget, 1958). Formal operational thinking allows the individual to think in terms of symbols—to think about and reflect upon his or her own mental states. The adolescent also acquires the ability to recognize possibilities as well as actualities and to construct ideals which are not tied to the concrete world of the here-and-now. Thus, the adolescent can mentally solve abstract, propositional, "as if" problems which younger children either ignore or are incapable of solving.

The significance of these characteristics of formal operations lies in the expansion and freedom of thought that they permit the adolescent as compared to the child. Because of the developing capacity for thinking in terms of possibilities and ideals, adolescents are able to envision alternatives in situations they face. An adolescent is, therefore, more likely than a child to suggest alternative arguments to many of the rules, guidelines, and points of view offered by parents and previously accepted as givens by the young child. The parents, omniscient and omnipotent in the eyes of the young child, are now seen as having "feet of clay." Baranowski (1978) has noted that this perception results in adolescents' attempting to influence the attitudes and behaviors of their parents to a greater extent than is common in childhood. The rule system of the family may thus come under challenge as it is viewed from the different and critical eyes of the young person in transition to adulthood.

There is a secondary outcome of this new expansion and freedom of thought resulting from the advent of formal operations. In childhood, the parent-child relationship is characterized by a partial dependency concerning the interchange of ideas, attitudes, and feelings. There is a flow of ideas, attitudes, and feelings from the parent to the child. The child tends to parrot the parents' ideas as if they were his own: "That's bad." "You're not supposed to do that." "God made everything." This similarity in thinking creates a symbiotic relationship that is reinforcing to the parents; for the child's verbalizations indicate that the parent has successfully socialized the child. With the adolescent's increasing capacity for independent conceptualization of ideas, attitudes, and feelings, this reinforcement—this symbiosis—begins to fade, adding to perceived stress in the parent-adolescent relationship.

Accommodating to these challenges often involves changing established attitudinal patterns and behaviors or compromising standards. If, for a variety of reasons, the family cannot adapt to the changes in its adolescent member, the family system becomes vulnerable to some degree of stress. The nature and extent of the stress experienced are discussed in more detail in a later section of this chapter.

Identity Formation

As one outcome of the maturing of thought processes, adolescents begin to take a different and more complex view of themselves. According to Erikson (1950, 1959, 1963, 1968), with the advent of pubescence there emerges the ego problem of articulating values, fantasies, and identification with ideals, plans, and expectations in the process of identity formation. Identity suggests being true to oneself as well as finding someone or something to be true to outside of oneself in order to prove one's capacity for fidelity. Developmental influences that contribute to the perception of oneself as distinct from others and as a reasonably consistent and continuous "whole" person contribute to a sense of ego identity. Any influences that impede this self-perception promote what Erikson has referred to as identity diffusion or role confusion, which is a failure to achieve an integration and overall continuity of self-image. The search for identity may lead an adolescent to adopt, at least temporarily, moral, religious, and political ideologies that are different from those of the parents.

James Marcia's (1966) research confirms and elaborates on Erikson's theory of identity formation. Marcia indicates that for the development of a mature and differentiated ego identity, it is necessary for the young person to question and challenge the existing familial value systems, goals, and beliefs with which they have been raised. This search is sometimes painful and often involves varying degrees of crises on the part of the adolescent. Consider, for example, a young man who has blindly accepted his parents' ambitions for him to follow in the family business. It was always expected that he would make the family proud by living up to parental expectations. The young person does not look within himself and challenge the appropriateness of this choice to his own values, ambitions, and self-perceptions. Foreclosing on a career decision without at least some degree of inner struggle leaves the person with an incomplete identity in that important area of life.

When a child attempts to depart from parental values, such as in adopting a different religious ideology, parents may react in a variety of ways. Some are challenged to rethink their own values; others may feel strongly concerned and wonder "where we went wrong"; still others, feeling threatened, may respond in an authoritarian manner by restricting activities of their adolescents to experiences that are compatible with the parental values. The latter situation may have serious implications. If parents insist on continual obedience to their values, the adolescent can either become rebellious or passively give lip service to the parental standards. In giving lip service, the youth may introject the parental demands into his or her own ego. When this happens, the achievement of a mature identity becomes difficult (Marcia, 1966).

Ackerman (1958) noted that there is a dynamic interrelation between the identity of the adolescent and the identity of the family unit. The challenges and changes common in the adolescent's search are often difficult to harmonize with a stable family identity. The adolescent's need for growth and autonomy and the parents' needs for maintenance and continuity of family structure may conflict with one another. This does not necessarily mean that there is serious conflict between parents and adolescents; however, it seems undeniable that the process of adolescent identity formation is experienced as stressful in some families.

There are two situations which further complicate the process of identity articulation in adolescence and hence contribute further to family stress. First is the wide number of options and choices available to adolescents in Western industrialized countries. The identity-in-formation is likely to be a confused one, as the adolescent confronts a wide variety of options in ideologies, careers and lifestyles from which to create a future.

The second situation concerns the definition of adulthood. The ultimate goal of adolescent growth and development is, of course, to become an adult as defined by the society. In American society there are many definitions of adulthood—biological, legal, societal, psychological. These produce confusion and frustration for the adolescent and for the parents who are attempting to cope with their adolescents' advances toward adulthood.

For example, from the biological perspective, adulthood is achieved when the young person attains reproductive capacity. Legal adulthood is achieved by attaining a certain age, an age which differs depending upon the activity. Driving a car, drinking alcohol, marrying, voting, entering into contracts—all have differing ages and these ages may vary from state to state. In the social realm, Erikson (1968, p. 265) wrote; "I have suggested that the mental and emotional ability to receive and give fidelity marks the conclusion of adolescence, while adulthood begins with the ability to receive and give love and care." Other writers (e.g., Havighurst, 1972; Komopka, 1973) seem to believe that adulthood begins when the psychosocial tasks of adolescence have been concluded. Levinson and his colleagues (1978) do not see adulthood as beginning until the early thirties, when the first integration of disparate elements of the self has taken place. Modell, Furstenberg, and Hershberg (1976) write that adulthood involves a number of psychosocial transitions which are accomplished over a span of years. Such variations in definition contribute to stress in the family. When has the adolescent become an adult?

In concluding this section, it is well to remember that, although this discussion focuses on modern industrialized society, the existence of tension between parents and adolescents brought about by qualitative changes in thinking and the quest for an individual identity is not a new phenomenon, as pointed out early in this paper. Among the hundreds of historical accounts of the conflict between adolescents and parents is one written by Simone de Beauvoir about her youth during the early 1900s:

I had lost the sense of security childhood gives, and nothing had come to take its place. My parents' authority remained inflexible, but as my critical sense developed I began to rebel against it more and more. I couldn't see the point of visits, family dinners, and all those tiresome social duties which my parents considered obligatory. Their replies . . . didn't satisfy me at all. My mother . . . had her own "ideas" which she did not attempt to justify, and her decisions often seemed to me quite arbitrary. We had a violent argument . . . (Kiell, 1964; p. 275).

PARENTAL DEVELOPMENT

In any discussion of the crisis-like development of an adolescent member of a family, it is necessary to include a perspective on the developmental stages of the other members of the family, especially in situations where the other members may be experiencing crises in their own development. It has been suggested that a "developmental crisis" of any family member can be viewed most meaningfully as a family crisis in that such periods of stress are reflective of or stimulate changes in the family group (Hadley, Jacob, Millones, Caplan, & Spitz, 1974).

More than two decades ago, McArthur (1962) gave a rather convincing argument that much of the parent-adolescent conflict could be explained by the fact that individual developmental tasks of adolescents come into direct opposition with the developmental tasks of their middle-aged parents. At the same time that the adolescent is going through a developmental crisis, the adult parents face developmental tasks as well.

More recently, Levinson et al. (1978) describe adulthood as consisting of relatively stable periods of approximately seven years punctuated by periods of transition, generally lasting five years. The transition years often are marked by turmoil, uncertainty, and a reawakening of issues unresolved in earlier years. Levinson et al. (1978) identified the years 28 to 33, 40 to 45, 50 to 55, and 60 to 65 as years of adult transitions. Stress theory would suggest that when the parents' transition periods coincide with offspring's transitions, the family system will undergo greater strain than when the parents' transition periods occur before or after the adolescence of their children.

Relationships between the generations should be smoother when parents feel productive, centered, in control of their lives. While outside events may shatter these feelings at any point in the life course, the transition periods appear to be those when inner events disrupt the adult's self-perceptions and sense of well-being. The presence in the home of an adolescent who questions parental values and customs may exacerbate the parents' own inner turmoil.

The adolescent unwittingly contributes to the parents' developmental crisis in other ways as well. Parents in mid-life often become aware of the child's budding sexual attractiveness and vigor at a time when they perceive their own sexual attractiveness to be waning. Reassessments in other areas of their lives are often triggered by the presence of youthful hope evidenced by an adolescent in the home. Career reassessments can lead to the realization that one's own career has reached a climax. The dream of becoming a great writer, a college president, or a foreman conflicts with the reality that one falls short of the mark set in younger days. A father may feel resentment toward a son who is "just starting" and for whom dreams and ideals remain possibilities. A mother may be resuming a career of her own or seeking ways of starting a career and may envy her daughter's opportunity to start early in life. As parents are coming to terms with sorting out their mistakes and the realities of their lives, adolescents have the hopes, dreams, imagination, opportunity, idealistic goals. The parent may feel envy and resentment; the adolescent may become impatient with limitations imposed by society and "conservative" parents. Thus, two generational transitions exist together—often feeding on each other—with the potential for at least a mild amount of stress.

A SYSTEMS PERSPECTIVE ON FAMILY COPING

In this section we attempt to give conceptual meaning in terms of systems theory to the stress affecting the family and its ability to cope during the adolescence of a family member. In order to make progress in understanding the role adolescents play in contributing to family stress, we must place our discussion within a relevant theoretical framework.

An overview of systems theory as it applies to the family is presented first. Some important concepts are defined which help us to understand stress in the parent-adolescent relationship. Also discussed are the various ways, both functional and dysfunctional, in which family members often respond to and cope with the stresses.

An Overview of Systems Theory

Systems theory is a model of reality which consists "fundamentally of relationships among relationships" (Ball, 1978, p. 66). A system "is a set of interacting units with relationships among them" (Miller, 1978, p. 281), and a family can be seen most meaningfully as such a system. The basic structure of a system places it within a boundary, namely the family unit. The family system has *input* (i.e., a stimulus received from the environment such as adding a new member, information, or income); family transformation of or *reactions to the input*; and *output*; (i.e., responses emitted by the family system to the environment such as solutions, information). Rules of transformation between the input and output of a family system govern change and stability in the family unit. In a process called morphogenesis, new rules of transformation may be introduced by the family system to meet the needs which are created by stressful new or novel situations (Broderick & Smith, 1979; Speer, 1970).

Coping: Feedback and Rules of Transformation

Broderick and Smith (1979, p. 115) have described four levels of feedback and system control: ". . . a system's capability to monitor its own progress toward a set goal, to correct and to elaborate its response, and even to change its goals depends upon the complexity of its feedback structure." Feedback to the system, the ability to perceive its output at one point as input at some subsequent point, is a particularly important process in the rules of transformation of a system. Rules of transformation tell the system what to do with feedback. Such rules are usually unspoken but are mutually understood.

The four levels of transformation which govern change and stability in a family system are now described in more detail. For example, when the degree of clutter in an adolescent's room reaches a parentally perceived critical level, i.e., the parent notices it, the "rule" may be to issue threats or bribes to the adolescent to clean it up. Alternatively, in some families, the rule may be that a parent or housekeeper has responsibility for the cleaning of all rooms. In either case, the stimulus, room clutter, provides an automatic response, to reduce clutter, i.e., to dampen the input. A *level 1* operation has been invoked.

To use the same example at *level 2*, the degree of the clutter, small amount, medium amount, huge amount, triggers a different response. With a small amount of clutter the rule may be to issue a simple request to the adolescent to pick things up. When the clutter is at a medium amount, a time-limit or small threat may be added to the request. However, a large amount of clutter may invoke a rule that directs the parent to immediately rescind privileges until the room is restored to a parentally approved appearance. At level 1 or 2 the success or failure of the rule is *not* evaluated. If the rule fails, stronger aspects of it may be invoked, but the rule is not changed.

At the *third level* of control, rules of transformation may be altered or changed; the system changes, rather than remaining in a steady state. Broderick and Smith believe that this change or morphogensis is a developmental phase of a system, undertaken when customary rules of transformation have failed to achieve system goals.

Thus, at level 3, the failure of a rule may lead to change in the rule. The parent's goal of an uncluttered room remains, but when a previous rule fails, the parent creates or finds a new rule to apply to the feedback that the adolescent's room is cluttered. For example, the rule described above which implied that the parent is responsible for alerting the child to the undesirable appearance of the room may give way to a new rule: Every Saturday morning is clean-up day.

At the *fourth level*, the system undergoes a conversion, or reorientation so that its goals change. Feedback presumably is used to ensure that the output meets the wholly new goals of the system. To continue with our example of the cluttered room, at level four, the goal of an uncluttered adolescent's room may be altered. The parent may conclude that as long as the door is closed it is up to the adolescent to regulate the level of clutter in the room. The parent's goal has changed. No longer is a neat room desired, only a closed door.

The differences among these four levels is that at level 1 feedback produces an automatic response; at level 2 feedback produces control on the output among several possibilities, which are still part of the existing rules of transformation; at level 3 feedback produces change in the system so that output includes possibilities which did not exist previously. All of these processes are in the service of unchanged fundamental system goals. Level 4 recognizes that systems goals may change.

The above discussion is summarized in Figure 1 below.

Goals remain the same			
Level 1	Level 2	Level 3	Level 4
Automatic response	A criterion is used to evaluate and shape response	Rules are evaluated	System undergoes a conversion
		Rules may change	Goals may change

Success or failure of a rule is not evaluated; rules remain unchanged

Figure 1. Levels of transformation in a family system which govern change and stability

It is important to recognize that all levels of operation are useful and potentially important for families as they develop throughout the life cycle; no level is inherently better than another. Level 3 and 4 operations are generally thought of as levels which result in growth and change. Obviously, however, a system which operates continuously at levels 3 and 4 in all activities would be in a constant state of turmoil, having to continuously evaluate and change. For instance, a father need not evaluate each night whether he turns off the lights in the house; it is an automatic response. Level 1 and 2 operations can promote stability in the family when rules bring the family back to the previous state (before input).

The process of growth in families often occurs when the system requires a reorganization. Change and growth levels may be triggered when there is a crisis or stress. This can result from externally induced crises or stressors, such as death, illness, or sudden economic collapse of a community; or internal stressors, such as the developmental transitions of one or more family members, as in adolescence or middle age. An adaptive, healthy family can operate successfully at all levels as needs and circumstances require.

FAMILY SYSTEMS AND THE ADOLESCENT

In analyzing the family with an adolescent from a systems perspective, one must examine the rules of transformation, both implicit and explicit, used to maintain the family system and provide for its growth. In a living system the components of the system—the parents and the children who make up the family—are not static; each is changing according to his or her own biological and social clock. Writing from a dialectic perspective, Riegel (1976) has described human development as simultaneous movement along at least four dimensions: inner-biological, inner-psychological, cultural-sociological, and outer-physical. Development is a process of leaps brought about by asynchrony, i.e., a lack of coordination among two or more of the four dimensions. Adding to Riegel's description, we suggest that when asynchrony occurs, a crisis in development is described which may produce growth or decay depending upon how the family system handles the crisis.

Adolescence is a stage of development characterized by asynchrony, or lack of coordination, in a number of areas. The adolescent may be well developed in the biological area, appear physically adult, and have the capacity to reproduce, but he/she may be in the early phases of development of those cognitive changes described earlier, during which the ability to reason and to make mature judgments fluctuates widely. These fluctuations remind the parent of a child at one moment and of an adult at another moment. Judged against the young person's adult appearance, the adolescent's behavior may appear "childlike," or worse, "adolescent."

The family system of parents with adolescent children is thus one which faces realignments of or shifts in relationships through the necessary developmental changes of its members. When a family member is undergoing a developmental crisis, as in adolescence, stress is often the result because previous patterns of rule transformation (i.e., the level of rule, the rule itself, or the goals) become inadequate. The family is forced to act. The rules for meeting stress along with the family's resources for implementing the rules will determine the nature and extent of the stresses experienced.

A family's operation at levels 1 and 2 is adaptive when the rule system is adequate. However, when there is dissonance or incongruence, the family's ability to operate at level 3 or level 4 becomes important for the long-range success of the system (see Figure 1). Family therapists should be able to achieve some progress with a family in which the rule system is confused by helping them to decide when and how to adapt its rules of transformation to accommodate the changing situations created by a member in transition.

Internal Inconsistencies

It is important to keep in mind that the rule systems established by a family may seem clear, workable, and relatively easily enforced when the children are younger. Establishing and maintaining workable rules may be much more challenging during the stage of adolescence, especially with regard to what may be considered adult concerns such as the use of drugs, sexual behavior, money matters, employability, use of automobiles, and other signs of independence and self-reliance. The family may have explicit rules for consequences, yet an implicit understanding of latitudes of enforcement.

This leads to an interesting phenomenon that may arise in a family in which there is an adolescent. Even if parents have clear and explicitly defined rules for maintaining stability in the family, it remains necessary to deal emotionally with the change in status of the adolescent/emerging adult. Dealing with the change in status can trigger internal inconsistencies in the parents' rule systems. These inconsistencies may come about because of unresolved issues in the parents' own adolescence, lack of understanding or resolution of their current stage of life, and/or confusion over being open to new ideas versus being cautious and conservative in order to better guide their children.

Take, for example, a family system which has functioned smoothly through many developmental stages of its growing children. The family is able to operate at all four levels of functioning as the need arises. This particular family prides itself on its openness and flexibility. In the area of sexuality, for instance, the parents have provided for open discussions of sexual behavior in young people. The message to the children was: "we want you to feel free to express your sexuality in an open, accepting atmosphere." Explicitly, then, they are open and accepting.

When their oldest daughter enters pubescence, she becomes sexually active. Faced with the behavior of their daughter engaging in sexual intercourse, an internal inconsistency in the parents' rule system is triggered. This inconsistency arises out of a variety of complex and usually unarticulated reasons. Perhaps the parents were raised to believe that sex is "dirty" but thought they had "overcome it," or perhaps they are currently sexually frustrated in their own lives. Or, as part of her mid-life self-reassessment, the mother may perceive that her days of sexually seductive powers are numbered. This can arouse strong feelings of jealousy over her daughter's fresh ability to seduce. Likewise, the father may be wishing he had spent more time "carousing" before he settled down, or he may lament losing the love and affection of his daughter to another male. These feelings, juxtaposed with the adolescent's behavior, range in intensity from very mild to very strong among different parents, but they are rarely neutral. The parents' motives often become emotional and irrational, and no new rules can be introduced to stabilize the system. Resorting to an inappropriate level of operation, they exert punishment and authoritarianism, forbidding their daughter to ever again see her boyfriend. Accusing her parents of being "hypocrites," the daughter is confused and becomes hostile and disobedient. Faced with this stress, the family system's stability is challenged.

As mentioned earlier, many aspects of adolescent development require the family to reorganize its usual rules of maintaining family stability—what works for smaller children does not usually work for adolescents. The changes with regard to formal operations and to identity formation are important examples. Thus, when an adolescent challenges the values, beliefs, and standards of the parents, there is a break in established agreements requiring reorganization of the rule system. When an adolescent announces to religious parents that he or she has become an agnostic, for example, it can be especially threatening to parents who do not understand the process of identity formation with its necessary challenges to established ways of thinking. If the parents' belief system is rigidly held in a closed-minded manner, then their response is usually to use a level 1 solution inappropriately. The family is unable to alter its established rule system with regard to religious beliefs, and the system comes under stress. For a healthy solution, the family is called upon to create new rules of handling this input to the system. If the parents are able to operate on a level of 3 or 4, they can either change their responses (e.g., learn to tolerate the challenge), change the guidelines for adolescent behavior (e.g., try to allow for more open discussions of religious beliefs), and/or even to change their goals. In any event, a response which *allows change* is most facilitative of the system's adaptation.

CONCLUSIONS AND IMPLICATIONS FOR TREATMENT AND POLICY

The systems perspective taken in this chapter has treated stress as not only inevitable, but necessary for growth and change. Interrelationships within the system may be stressful due to the developmental changes of the system members, the characteristic interaction of the family members, and/or the structure of the family system. When stress arises from the inevitable developmental changes of family members, the family that copes is the one which find strategies for dealing with these changes. The adolescent must eventually leave home to become an independent adult (Haley, 1980).

Throughout the adolescent years the interrelationships of the adolescent and the parents must be oriented to the inevitable system change. If the family fails to make rules of transformation which allow for change and for growth, the stress on the system will be more destructive than for systems which incorporate such rules in their functioning. Paradoxically, the system which can let go of its members is the system which will endure and reproduce itself effectively in later generations.

The stress which has been discussed in this chapter is normative in nature, rather than pathological. A family experiencing such stress is unlikely to require professional intervention for corrective treatment. However, it is desirable for adolescents, families, and communities to understand the stress often inherent in developmental transitions, their sources, and their possible outcomes. Thus, primary and secondary *prevention* constitutes the most basic intervention strategies.

Secondary preventive intervention exists in the form of transitory counseling of the family, delivered under the auspices of churches, schools, and counseling professionals. Thus, intervention for secondary prevention is available wherever there are churches and schools. The mechanism for primary intervention, however, is not institutionalized.

In the modern world, scientists/professionals have not achieved a balance between roles as scientists and as professional counselors or teachers. Even with the institutional supports that exist, there are few prevention-oriented delivery systems or programs for relating to the community as a whole continuously over the years. Only when developmental problems become severe or are exacerbated do they receive attention.

To achieve primary *prevention* of serious distress in families with adolescents, the communications media may ultimately provide the needed social structure, perhaps in combination with policy decisions. The dissemination of information, replete with examples of a systems perspective, may prove particularly helpful to families of an adolescent or young adult. Understanding implicit and explicit family rules, perceiving not just alternative rules, but alternative ways of thinking about rules, should lead to reduced stress and more effective family functioning. In addition, any such educational program should provide explication of the developmental changes of both adolescents and adults and should highlight the stressful implications of these for families, particularly when developmental transitions occur simultaneously. It is our view that the stress of transitions can lead to enhanced growth of the family, and all of its members, and to possibilities for rewarding interactions among vital and healthy individuals.

6

Dual-Career Families: Strains of Sharing

DENISE A. SKINNER

Susan Higgins tries to leave her law office by 5:30 p.m., so she'll have time to swing by the grocery store before picking up ten-year-old Michael and three friends from soccer practice at his school. She drops off the three friends at their homes and stops at the pharmacy to pick up some cough medicine for six-year-old Andrew. During the day she had called the pediatrician about his lingering cold.

Susan hopes that Ron, her husband, will get to Andrew's afterschool day-care program by 5:30. Ron is director of a large community social services agency, and is often delayed by end of the day problems. If he is late again, the day-care staff will be annoyed. But when she and Michael get home at 6:15, Ron is making dinner, and Andrew is dawdling at setting the table.

Dinner is almost the only time the family has to talk together, so Susan and Ron devote all their attention to the boys' stories of the day or their interest in the latest TV show. Right after dinner, Ron

This project was funded by a grant from the Agricultural Experiment Station, University of Minnesota. The author would like to thank Dr. Richard Sauer, Director, Agricultural Experiment Station, and Dean Keith McFarland, College of Home Economics, for their support.

rushes out to a county welfare committee meeting, and Susan settles into an evening of washing dishes, folding laundry, and helping the boys with homework. After they are in bed, she pulls out some paperwork. Ron gets home at 11 p.m. and the two finally have a few minutes for each other.

Both Susan and Ron know the demands for their careers and their family life mean both sacrifices and satisfactions. Susan sometimes feels guilty that she may be neglecting her sons, and occasionally resents the fact that, although Ron and the boys help out around the house, she still bears most of the responsibility for housework and child care. Ron wistfully recalls the days when Susan stayed at home with the children when they were small; even though they had less money and could not afford vacations or the twice-a-month cleaning service, they had more time to relax together. Also he feels ambivalent, sometimes jealous, over her commitment to her career; last year he turned down a better job in another state because she could not move at the time. Both Susan and Ron wish for more time and energy to spend together. But, on the satisfaction side, they both love their work, and the money they earn allows them to own a nice house, to send their children to good schools, and to share a lot of little luxuries. Susan feels more confident and assertive since she has returned to work, and both she and Ron feel this has strengthened their marriage.

Susan and Ron are part of a growing family form—the dual-career family. U. S. Department of Labor statistics reveal that the married female is a key source of growth in the rate of participation of women in the labor force, with over half of all wives now employed. These dual-worker families, those in which both wives and husbands are employed, are becoming commonplace for at least a portion of most families' life cycle. In such families the majority of the women (and many of the men) work in what might be called *jobs*, positions that are not a major life interest and are undertaken primarily to provide family income. However, there is a developing minority of families in which both the husband and wife pursue *careers* while maintaining a family life together. The word "career" is used here to refer to occupations which require a high degree of commitment and have a continuous developmental character (Rapoport & Rapoport, 1976). An individual typically pursues a career by obtaining education and relevant experience which enables him or her to perform with expertise. Career people tend to view their careers as a primary source of personal satisfaction. Dual-career families, then, are a subtype of the larger category of dual-worker families. We can assume that they have a great deal in common.

Why do dual-career families present a special interest? Such families, while still a minority pattern, are increasing in prevalence. As more and more women seek increased education and training, as sex roles become more flexible and sex-role equality continues to be emphasized, as the increased cost of living necessitates two incomes, the number of the dual-career families will, in all likelihood, increase.

However, a significant feature of the dual-career lifestyle is that it is associated with considerable stress and strain. The often competing demands of the occupational structure and those of a full family life present a number of challenges for dual-career family members. Much of the literature implies that the stress is inherent in a dual-career lifestyle. However, some of the constraints of the lifestyle might be explained by the fact that it is a relatively new and minority pattern. It has not been a national pattern for married women to work, much less to pursue careers. Rather, our society has had as a dominant lifestyle a "conventional pattern" characterized by husbands as wage earners and wives as homemakers. Obviously, the dual-career lifestyle is "out of sync" with the pattern and the social structure and mores which support conventional family living. This can result in stress for dual-career family members. In meeting the challenges of the dual-career lifestyle, couples have been forced to come up with individualized solutions, as very few societal supports exist (Holmstrom, 1973).

Therefore, it seems important for family professionals as well as couples considering dual-career living to understand the special challenges it presents. The purpose of this chapter is to contribute to this understanding by: (a) describing the sources of stress in dual-career living; (b) discussing the impact of such strains on various family members, and (c) presenting the resources and coping strategies utilized by dual-career families in managing their lifestyles.

DUAL-CAREER STRESSORS

Although there is considerable variation from one family to another in the types of stressors experienced and the ways in which they impact on dual-career family members, there are also common patterns. Rhona and Robert Rapoport, pioneers in the field of dual-career family research, have identified a number of dilemmas of the dual-career family which by their nature set up strains. An adaptation of their findings is presented below.

Overload

The problem of work and role overload is a common source of stress for dual-career families. The responsibilities of two careers, children, a marriage, and a home are considerable and demand most, if not all, of the time and energy of dual-career couples. These individuals often report "racing against the clock," being "involved in a continual juggling act" as they attempt to keep in balance their many roles. While couples deal differently with the overload problem, it is quite common for many to use money to help alleviate some of the strain. Hiring help, especially for child-care, is a common expense in this lifestyle. Couples also "buy time" in various other ways, such as hiring outside help to do domestic work and purchasing labor and time-saving items (e.g., microwave ovens and "no-iron" clothing).

Other dual-career families attempt to reorganize household roles, with the husband and children taking on more of what traditionally has been the wife's responsibility. However, it appears that in many families the wife still assumes the major responsibility for domestic tasks (Bryson, Bryson, & Johnson, 1978; Holmstrom, 1973; Paloma, 1972; Rapoport & Rapoport, 1976).

Identity and Normative Issues

These stresses stem from traditional sex-role socialization and stereotyping, which suggest that men "should" be occupationally successful, powerful, in command, etc. and that women "should" be skilled in cooking and other domestic activities, nurturing, passive, and deferring to men. Such internalized values from early socialization often create ambivalence, guilt, self-doubt and tension for dual-career couples attempting more egalitarian roles.

Couples utilize a variety of behaviors in coping with identity and normative dilemmas. Most couples define their dual-career pattern as favorable or advantageous to them and their families when compared to other alternatives available; in doing so, they reduce some psychological strain. For instance, many career mothers remind themselves that they are happier mothers and wives when working outside the home than they would be if they were fulltime homemakers. Some females also report attempting to segregate work and family roles as much as possible. They purposely leave their work, expertise, and status at the office at the end of the day, enabling them to perform in their self- and family-defined roles as wife and mother. As one woman commented, "When I hang up my lab coat at the end of the day I try to hang up any work-related issues with it. As I drive home, I make the transition from medical researcher to wife and mother."

Compromise is a common coping strategy in reducing the psychic strain associated with identity and normative issues. Women in particular compromise career goals if there are competing role demands (Epstein, 1971; Heckman, Bryson, & Bryson, 1977; Holmstrom, 1973). However, some males in dual-career families make career sacrifices also, e.g., compromising advancement opportunities in order that their wives may continue in their careers, as Ron Higgins did, or turning down a promotion because the advancement would mean increased time demands on his already time-deficient family.

Finally, dual-career couples report that friendships with other dual-career couples are helpful supports to them. In such instances each could validate the other's lifestyle and provide an empathetic support structure.

Role-Cycling and Scheduling Issues

The dilemma of role-cycling refers to attempts by the dual-career couple to mesh the demands of their individual career cycles with the changing responsibility of the different family life cycle stages. Generally, the most stressful times occupationally are when the individual is establishing himself or herself on the job and again when one is promoted or assumes new or added responsibilities. Similarly, various time periods in the family, such as the childbearing stage and adolescence of the children have been noted to be particularly stressful. Many dual-career couples attempt to avoid additional strain by staggering their career and family cycles so that peak career and family stress times are not occurring simultaneously. For this reason, such couples establish themselves occupationally before having children.

The complexity of coordinating daily schedules is also a concern of most dual-career family members. Because they are meshing *two* daily occupational schedules with individual family members' schedules, dual-career couples are very conscious of how they spend their time. Jobs which give the individual flexibility in controlling his or her schedule are highly valued in such families, as it makes it much easier to meet family obligations, such as getting the children to their dental appointments. Dual-career individuals report having to organize their time and efforts carefully, relying heavily on lists and calendars.

It is not uncommon for such couples to carefully schedule "family time" (e.g., "From the time I get home until the children go to bed is their time") or time alone as a couple in order to insure that these important relationships receive the attention the couple desires for them. Many couples report that there is simply not time for everything and that certain activities are forfeited in order to have time to accomplish things higher on their priority list.

Entertaining in one's home, leisure time alone, and participation in community activities are examples of just a few of the activities career couples report engaging in less frequently than others.

Career Demands

There are many aspects of the occupational milieu which make it difficult to have two careers in one family. As Holmstrom (1973, p. 29) pointedly noted: "The trouble with having a profession today is that if you have one, you are expected to pursue it in a certain way—and it is a very rigid way." First of all, there are stringent expectations as to how a career is to be pursued. The demand for single-minded continuous commitment required by most careers is a potential stressor for many families and particularly for dual-career families. Such an orientation may assume that other family members' needs will be subordinated to the career and that a "support person" (typically the wife) will be available for entertaining, managing the home, and caring for the children. It also often means that an "interrupted" career pattern characterized by part-time employment will be judged less favorably when it comes to hiring and promotions.

The demands for occupational mobility and immobility presents another barrier for dual-career families (Holmstrom, 1973). Some jobs require moves by the individual in order to retain the position or to be promoted. Although there are increasing numbers of high-ranking employees who are refusing job transfers, career development is still generally enhanced if one is able to be mobile.

The opposite of mobility is important also. Sometimes it is necessary to stay put in a certain location long enough to finish an education or establish oneself in a specific profession. It is to the individual's advantage to be able to do this without having to consider the occupational needs of other family members.

Obviously, in the dual-career family, the situation is more complex. Dual-career couples report that their spouse's career influences their decision about where to live in varying degrees. In Holmstrom's study (1973) of two-career couples, every wife reported that her decision about where to live was significantly influenced by her husband. Often the couples negotiated simultaneously for a set of positions and sometimes the wife followed the husband. In some instances, the wife wanted to move but was restricted to one place because her husband could not, or would not, move. In the majority of couples, the husband's decision about where to live was, also, significantly influenced by his wife's career. In such instances, the couples negotiated for a set of positions, considering the needs of both partners, and for a few couples, the husband followed the wife.

Some couples solve the mobility issue by deciding to live apart for periods ranging from a few days each week to months at a time in order to pursue their respective careers. Called "commuter," "long-distance," or "two-location" families, these couples maintain two separate homes, reuniting at established times. While this living arrangement may solve the stress that would be experienced if one or the other partner were not able to pursue his or her career, it may create other stressors. The expenses of this lifestyle (travel, telephone bills, two residences) are a burden for most of these families. Couples also report missing the everyday routines (sharing daily experiences, eating meals together, sitting quietly together) that produces the ordered world typically entailed in a marital relationship (Geretal & Gross, 1981).

The rigidity of the occupational structure, then, serves as a major barrier for dual-career couples. Some dual-career couples are, in an *ad hoc* manner, negotiating work arrangements which will reduce or remove some of this stress. Flexible scheduling, job sharing, and split-location employment are utilized by dual-career couples lucky enough to have employers who provide flexible work policies.

EFFECTS OF STRAIN

The potential sources of strain discussed above suggest that the stress a dual-career family experiences may be considerable. In examining the impact of such strain one must consider the particular family characteristics, as well as the occupational situation. The presence (and number) or absence of children, as well as the stage of the family life cycle, affects the complexity of dual-career family living. One study of dual-career couples found that it was the older professional couples and those who had not had children who experienced the lifestyle most positively (Heckman, Bryson, & Bryson, 1977). The demands of childbearing, particularly the problems associated with finding satisfactory child-care arrangements, are reported as quite stressful by couples (especially the woman) in the childbearing stage of the family life cycle. Dual-career couples tend to have smaller families than the average. Realizing that the more children in the family the greater the complexity as well as time and energy commitments, these couples tend to limit their family size in order to manage both career and family.

What do we know about the effect of the various stressors on the wife, the husband, the marriage, and the children in dual-career families?

Wives

Most of the research conducted on dual-career families reports that the impact of the stress is felt most by women. Perhaps this is because a man can combine a professional career and parenting more easily than a woman because our culture expects less of a man with regard to familial responsibilities (Bernard, 1974).

Overload strain is a significant issue for many dual-career women. While many studies indicate that husbands and children *help* with household tasks more in dual-career families, when compared to conventional families, it is still the wife and mother who assumes the major household responsibilities. As one mother commented, "Even though my family helps with the actual household tasks, I'm the one who organizes what needs to be done when, and carries a mental list around in my head of what supplies we do or do not have in the cupboard. Juggling all of this with all of my job responsibilities sometimes requires more energy than I have."

Occupationally, it has been the woman who more often takes the risks, sacrifices more, and compromises career ambitions in attempting to make the dual-career lifestyle a manageable one. However, the majority of these women report that they are willing to tolerate these inequities as long as they can have both their career and family.

Husbands

Life for the dual-career male is not without its periods of stress, although the impact does not appear to be as significant as that reported for women. In a study commissioned by General Mills (1981), "a lack of time with family/children" and "less time to see each other" were the most frequently reported strains for men in dual-employed families. Another study which compared men in conventional and dual-career families found that the husbands of working wives were less satisfied with work, marriage, and life than husbands of non-working wives. One explanation for these findings may be that the dual-career husband loses part of his active support system when the wife is no longer functioning as fulltime homemaker. Furthermore, out of a sense of fairness, the husband may be assuming a greater share of housekeeping tasks which have not been valued highly in our culture.

The Marriage

Finding the time and energy to devote to maintaining and developing the marital relationship is a common dilemma of dual-career couples. A career woman spoke to one aspect of this dilemma when she commented, "Both my husband and I have very demanding careers. We each come home at the end of the day drained of energy, wanting to be waited on and taken care of. Presently, things seem to balance out but if we had children, I don't know how we would meet all the demands." Time alone as a couple is generally a precious commodity for dual-career couples with children.

Many of these couples also struggle with putting into practice their ideological preferences for an egalitarian marriage. As one young husband admitted, "It is much easier to *talk* about the equal sharing of work and family responsibilities than it is to actually carry it out."

Most dual-career husbands and wives each make considerable compromises in order that the other may pursue a career. Because of this, if each does not accept the high value the other places on career pursuit, conflict is inevitable (Rice, 1979). However, overinvolvement in one's career can result in marital strain, according to Ridley (1973), who concluded that tension in the marital relationship may occur when either partner becomes so highly involved in a job that family obligations are excluded.

Another potential source of marital strain often mentioned in relation to dual-career marriages is the issue of competitiveness. Certainly if the two partners are engaged in a continuous competitive rivalry, the relationship will very likely be strained. The Holmstrom (1973) study of dual-career couples reported that most of these couples did not feel competitive toward each other. Holmstrom has suggested that we begin looking at the issue of competition in a different way. She has pointed out that people may be placed "in competition" and not "feel competitive" and that, likewise, not being allowed to be in a situation of competition will not necessarily prevent competitive feelings. In the latter instance, it might be the conventional wife who has not entered the occupational world (which has been more valued in our society) who feels upset over not even getting to play the game.

Children

A crucial concern that many people have is what the effects are on the children when both parents are employed. The response to this issue is that there are many other, more important variables that contribute to the child's health and development than whether or not both parents work. Such factors include the overall quality of the family and marital relationships, the mother's attitude about and satisfaction with her employment, the husband's attitude about his wife working, etc.

Actually, dual-career couples may increase the degree of strain they themselves experience in an attempt to prevent the lifestyle from creating strain for their children. For instance, a couple may continually postpone going out alone as a couple or with other adult friends because of their sense of responsibility to their children. There is no evidence to suggest that the dual-career lifestyle, in and of itself, is stressful for the children. What may be more significant for the children is the degree of stress experienced by the parents, which may indirectly affect the children. In her study of maternal employment, Hoffman (1974) concluded that:

. . . the working mother who obtains satisfaction from her work, who has adequate arrangements so that her dual role does not involve undue strain, and who does not feel so guilty that she overcompensates is likely to do quite well, and under certain conditions, better than the nonworking mother (p. 142).

COPING METHODS

Although coping behaviors specific to the various stressors were discussed earlier, there is more to say about the general patterns of coping in dual-career families. Family stress theory suggests that the way family members define their situation is an important component influencing the impact of various stressors on the family (Burr, 1973). Applied to dual-career families, it appears that while acknowledging the strains they experience, these couples also view their lifestyle as the best of the alternatives available to them. Such couples are quick to point out the advantages of dual-career living—things like personal fulfillment, higher standard of living, pride in each other's accomplishments, providing desirable role models for their children, etc. The goal is to maintain an optimistic definition of their lifestyle, believing in its value for them.

Coping patterns which maintain, strengthen, and restructure the family system are important in dual-career living. Working out a "fair" schedule of household tasks for all family members and specifically planning family activities for all to do together are two examples of behaviors dual-career family members engage in to restructure and strengthen the family.

Family members also need to have a repertoire of behaviors which enable them to manage the psychological tensions and strains. Coping behaviors which allow them to attend to personal needs (e.g., jogging, relaxation activities) and those which focus on reducing the demands of the present situation (e.g., lowering standards for "how well" household tasks must be done) are vitally important.

A pattern of coping which attempts to accommodate family to work and work to family is evident and necessary in most dual-career families. For instance, career men and women may modify their work schedules, reducing the amount of time spent at work or working different hours in order to meet family needs. School teachers who plan for the birth of their children during summer months are attempting to accommodate major changes at home to their work requirements.

Finally, a coping pattern which involves obtaining support from outside the family, in terms of both interpersonal relationships and goods and services, is helpful to the dual-career family. Having empathetic friends with similar values can be a real source of support for dual-career family members. Women, in particular, seem to see this support as very important. Likewise, being able to purchase goods and services, using modern equipment, and eating out frequently are just some of the ways dual-career couples "buy time" and, thus, reduce overload stress.

Management of the dual-career lifestyle seems to call for an orchestrated response utilizing the various coping patterns in a balanced manner. Adaptive dual-career coping, then, involves the ability to attend to family needs, promote family equity, and establish a healthy balance between work and family. It also calls for managing tensions, believing in the value of the lifestyle, and developing an outside support system.

CONCLUSION

The focus of this chapter, the stresses of dual-career family living, might make one ask why anyone would choose this lifestyle! Increasingly, however, people *are* choosing dual-career living, a trend that will no doubt continue in the future. The perceived advantages of the lifestyle coupled with social trends promoting equality for men and women in marriage and in the occupational realm make dual-career living a choice of more and more couples.

Certainly this lifestyle presents special challenges and strains which must be considered. At present, our society provides very few collective solutions to aid dual-career couples in managing these stressors. Societal and occupational changes, such as flexible scheduling, increased availability of part-time employment, better group care for children, maternity and paternity leaves, would certainly help ameliorate some of the struggles of dual-career families. Meanwhile, those considering the dual-career lifestyle must deal with society as it is presently structured.

Couples who manage a dual-career lifestyle successfully might well be characterized as being flexible, willing to share power in their relationships, respectful of each other's right to self-fulfillment, willing to compromise in order to achieve equity in marriage, and free from rigid sex-role behavior. Those considering such a lifestyle for themselves should scrutinize their attitudes towards men's and women's roles and examine their ambitions and expectations about marriage, family, and work. Continuous commitment to a demanding career along with an active family life may require a high level of energy and also limit the amount of free time one has for spontaneous leisure activities. In other words, for most people undertaking this lifestyle, choices must be made and priorities set. While this may be acceptable for one person, another might find it stressful.

Women and men in the career planning stage of their lives who want a career, marriage (to a career person), and children can begin to plan taking all three goals into account. Furthermore, when getting married one should definitely discuss with one's partner these feelings and hopes for job, home, and family, for the dual-career lifestyle is indeed not only manageable but satisfying to a growing number of couples who have learned to cope well with the special challenges it presents.

7

Divorce:
Before, During, and After

CONSTANCE AHRONS

Elaine and Dick Burke have been married for 15 years and have three children. Elaine has been feeling depressed for the past two years and entered into individual therapy after first trying to deal with her depression on her own for a year. In the course of therapy she came to realize that her relationship with Dick was a major cause of her depression. Upon locating the source of her distress, she became more anxious and upset and looked for other solutions for her unhappy feelings. For example, she thought if they bought a new house, perhaps there would be fewer problems.

As she struggled with her feelings over the next year, the arguments increased between her and Dick. The children became more aware that their parents were unhappy and Timmy, their youngest child, aged nine, began to wet his bed. Both parents began to blame each other for causing Timmy to be so upset. As Elaine and Dick began to fight more, divorce became an option that they openly argued about. The arguments were followed by more reasonable discussion about the possibility of physically separating for a while.

Several months later, after a bad fight with Elaine, Dick moved out of the house. He thought that if he moved out until things "cooled down," they could work things out.

After two months of living apart, both Dick and Elaine were upset and lonely and decided to try living together again. Following a month of living together it was clear that nothing in their relationship had changed and Elaine and Dick began seriously discussing divorce and shared their feelings and decision with the children.

Then they separated, this time with some plans for how they would continue to manage the children, finances, and other issues and tasks. During the next year, Dick, Elaine, and the children went to a family therapist to help them work out communication problems about the children (e.g., differences in discipline in each of their households).

After about six counseling sessions they were able to draw up a contract that spelled out many of these issues (i.e., who the children would spend which vacations with, who would be in charge of the children's allowances, how they would decide on summer camp). The therapist helped them define their new relationship as coparents (the parenting relationship between divorced parents) and to view themselves as a family—a binuclear family. They realized that, although their binuclear family was very different from their married nuclear family—in that there were now two households—they were still a family. Although Elaine and Dick decided on joint custody of the children, the two younger children had their primary residence with Elaine and the older child had his primary residence with Dick. This child-care arrangement was to remain flexible so that living arrangements would depend on the developmental needs of the children and the wishes of the parents.

Although Elaine and Dick were still angry with each other, they were able to structure and shorten their conversations to focus on the children's needs. The only occasions that the binuclear family spent together were "one-time situations" (e.g., when Timmy received an award at a Boy Scout dinner). Both Elaine and Dick had independent lives and interacted with each other only when it was necessary to discuss an issue related to the children.

This whole process took five years. If and when either Dick or Elaine remarry, they will need to expand their family system to include a stepparent, which will probably create some initial distress as the family adapts to a new member.

As divorce rates continue to rise in the United States, more and more people will spend time as a part of a divorced family at some time in their lives. The child of divorced parents who both remarry may have two biological parents, two stepparents, biological siblings, step and half siblings, up to eight grandparents, and any number of additional extended relatives through the new spouses of the biological parents. Imagine the confusion such a child might experience—and the stigma he or she might feel when attempting to describe this family in school. Our culture lacks the concepts and kinship terms to describe such a complex network of interrelationships in the divorced family. Given the current divorce and remarriage rates, a rough projection is that about one-fourth of all children growing up today will experience this new extended family and will have more than two parents before they reach age 18 (Furstenberg, 1979).

Because divorce touches so many people—adults as well as children—and because it is important to reduce feelings of shame and confusion, it is helpful to think of divorce as a normative family transition and not a sign of a "bad" or "failed" family. This is not to say that divorce is not a stressful process; like other family transitions it can bring unhappiness and always requires adjustment.

In this chapter we will review some of the numerous reports and studies of the effects of divorce on the family and put forward the concept of the binuclear family as a useful family model. Then, using the case example of the Burke family, we will review the stressors associated with each transition or phase in the divorce process, suggesting functional and dysfunctional coping patterns at each phase.

REEXAMINING THE STRESSFUL EFFECTS OF
DIVORCE: TOWARDS A NORMATIVE
DEFINITION

Studies conducted during the past 25 years make it abundantly clear that divorce has, for the most part, been regarded as a sign of social disorder; most writers and researchers have focused on the causes of marital separation rather than the consequences (Kitson & Raschke, 1981). Much of the literature which does focus on consequences deals with the effect of divorce on children.

Effects of Divorce on Children

The existing literature on the effects of divorce on children (e.g., Goldstein, Freud, & Solnit, 1973; Westman, 1972) tends to emphasize the "maladjusted" behavior of children. This focus gives rise to and perpetuates a distorted perception of divorce. Findings from these clinical studies conclude that divorce inevitably leads to family instability. This view is reflected in the terms used in our society to describe the structure of the divorced family: "broken home," "disorganized," "fractured," "incomplete," and the like.

To read these studies is to conclude that divorce is potentially a major stressor on children, especially young children. But a more careful examination suggests that it is not the divorce itself that produces psychological stress but rather specific hardships and demands that can result from divorce. The two most important hardships are (a) the absence of the father from both the home and a continuing relationship with his child; and (b) the continuance of conflict between parents, particularly during the period following the legal divorce.

No broad generalizations can be made about the effect of father absence on children (Herzog & Sudia, 1973; Luepnitz, 1978). A major methodological problem with most of this literature is the failure to consider the degree and duration of father absence. For example, does it make a difference if the father never sees the children, sees them only once a year, or once a month? If he continues to be interested in their lives or not? This critical omission in the research is probably generated by the underlying assumption that divorce *per se* inevitably leads to total family dissolution. The father who does not have custody of his children is ignored and automatically considered outside of the family. Almost all of the research conducted before 1976 could be relabeled studies on the effects of "father loss" on children's development.

Research studies of the effects of continued conflict between parents are less tentative in their conclusions: Conflict between parents causes severe psychological stress on children. Again, it is important to note that it is the conflict and not the divorce itself which produces the stress.

Normalizing Divorce

The high incidence of divorce in our country requires that we conceptualize divorce in terms of a model that does not regard it as an indication of abnormality and emotional instability. Divorce can be conceptualized as a *normative* family transition or change. It may be seen as a transition like many other normal family changes, such as a death in the family; divorce, like other transitions, can bring unhappiness to families, and it does demand a change in family structure, rules, and roles. These changes, however, do not mean that the divorced family is "bad" or "sick." Divorce may be seen as a process which involves the change or expansion of the traditional nuclear family (or mother, father, and children) from living in one residence to what may be termed a binuclear family. The binuclear family still includes both biological parents, even though they live apart. If either or both parents remarry, then the binuclear family also includes stepparents and step/half siblings. The divorced system, in which both parents continue to be part of the child's family, can help to reduce the stress of the divorce. The child does not have to lose either parent; nor is one parent burdened with the role of "single parent," for as coparents they can continue to share the responsibilities of childrearing (Ahrons, 1979, 1980b, 1980c).

TRANSITIONS OF THE DIVORCE PROCESS: STRESSORS AND COPING STRATEGIES

Unlike family crises of sudden onset, the divorce process begins long before the actual decision to obtain a legal divorce. Unlike war or death, in which external causes separate marriage partners, divorce is an internal crisis of relationship. It is a deliberate dissolution of the primary bond in the family, and the family's identity can appear shattered.

In this section we will use the case example from the beginning of the chapter to examine five transitions in the divorce process. The stressors involved at each stage as families adjust to changes in roles and the functional and dysfunctional coping strategies family members use will be examined. The five transitions are: (a) individual cognition; (b) family metacognition; (c) separation; (d) family reorganization; and (e) family redefinition.

These five stages describe a process during which family members take on new roles and the family itself takes on a new definition. Role changes are major sources of stress throughout the process; not only must parents adopt new roles as former spouses, but they also must adjust to a new parenting situation. The children in turn must learn to adjust to being cared for by their mother and father in a different way. Further complicating this process, however, is the social ambiguity surrounding the divorce and postdivorce family roles. It can be argued that the lack of clear role models for divorcing couples contributes to a higher amount of crisis. McCubbin (1979) suggests that the family's vulnerability to stress is influenced by the clarity of community expectations and norms. Given the role ambiguity for the divorced in our culture, the divorcing family is in a highly vulnerable state.

Transition I: Individual Cognition

For Elaine and Dick, Elaine's depression was the first sign that something was wrong. It took her some time to realize she was feeling depressed because of her marriage; even then she looked for a solution less drastic than divorce, such as buying a new house. Her individual cognition was the first stage in the divorce process. Characteristic of the dysfunctional coping mechanisms in the first stage of the divorcing process—individual cognition—is the denial of marital problems (Weiss, 1976; Wiseman, 1975).

Depression in one of the spouses or children is a common response to marital distress; Elaine and Dick's son also experienced emotional problems. Spouses also resort to blaming in order to obtain respite from a situation perceived as intolerable. The marital conflict escalates and the search for the fault in the other spouse often results in his or her being labeled the culprit. This time can be a highly stressful one, especially for the children, who often become pawns in the marital strife. Partners used to conflict may find it less threatening to stay with spouse than to face the uncertainty and change that accompanies separation and divorce. However these highly conflictual "intact" marriages appear more damaging to children's psychological and emotional development than the disorganization associated with divorce (Lamb, 1977; Magrab, 1978).

The type of resolution chosen during this transition may vary with the couple's history of coping patterns (Hansen & Hill, 1964). They frequently decide the best resolution is to delay divorce until a less disruptive time. For example, they will decide to stay in the marriage until the kids are grown. Other coping strategies include the decision to spend time and energy on interests outside the family while attempting to maintain the façade of an intact marriage. This process of emotional divorce, the withdrawal of emotional investment in the marital relationship, is self-protective and may have some positive benefits for the individual, although this withdrawal will reverberate throughout the family system.

The duration of this transition depends on the coping behaviors employed and other factors related to the family's vulnerability to stress. Equilibrium in the family is usually maintained, although precariously, during this transition. Role patterns may remain undisrupted despite the growing tension in the family. Families may deal with internal stress by assigning one member the role of family scapegoat, who is then blamed for causing trouble (Vogel & Bell, 1968). In this first stage, then, many of the coping strategies families use to alleviate feelings about the parents' marital difficulties often heighten stress in the family.

Transition II: Family Metacognition

The second transition is when the family as a whole begins to share the realization that the marriage is disintegrating. Family metacognition is family stocktaking; "metacognition" simply means that the family system begins to change in recognition of the problem. Elaine and Dick reached this stage when they began to talk seriously about separating and when they discussed their decision with the children.

At this stage, family members more or less openly discuss the situation and realize the problem (Flavell, 1979). This exchange of information sums up each family member's anxieties; the family recognizes the problem, its potential solutions, and its consequences. If the family can cope well enough to survive this transition, a physical separation of the spouses will occur. This time can be used to prepare for the changes caused by physical separation without making decisions based on anger. If the family has not employed a rational, sequential method of problem-solving in past crises, however, it is not apt to do so at this time. Due to the persistent emotional bonds between spouses, regardless of quality, this period is marked by ambivalent feelings of love and hate, euphoria and sadness (Weiss, 1976).

For some families this is the time of greatest disequilibrium. Husband and wife roles are fading, but new ones (i.e., divorced coparents) have not yet developed. The future appears ambiguous, and the family searches for role models. In striving for stability, the family may try to preserve old rules and rituals, only to realize that old patterns fail to provide comfort or unity. Children often begin to seek information about divorce by consciously looking for friends whose parents are divorced.

Transition III: Separation

There are great variations in family coping patterns during the third transition, separation, when one partner moves out of the family. The degree of crisis depends on how well family members have adjusted to the realization that the marriage has come to an end.

Couples commonly engage in a long transition of separation, as Elaine and Dick did; in many families, parents separate and reconcile briefly, because of feelings of ambivalence or guilt over the children's distress. Both Elaine and Dick felt lonely and unhappy during their first period of separation, and so were willing to try living together again.

The stress in families during these intermittent periods of separation and reconciliation may resemble the stress experienced by wives of military personnel missing in action, (Boss, 1977) and corporate wives (Boss, McCubbin, & Lester, 1979). Like these families, the family in separation is in a state of flux, and family members may be in doubt about new family roles and boundaries. A child might wonder if his parents are both still part of his family. In the most common divorced family form, mother and children remain as one unit, while father moves out and functions as a separate unit. The mother-headed household faces a dilemma: Should it reorganize and fill roles enacted by the physically absent father, or should it maintain his psychological presence in the system by not reorganizing? If the mother/children unit tries to reassign roles, the father's return will be met with resistance. This is what Boss (1977) refers to as boundary ambiguity. If, on the other hand, they deal with father as psychologically present, they perpetuate family disequilibrium and stress. This cycle is typical of the stress endured during this period. The children face a difficult and very stressful transition if the family remains in a state of disequilibrium characterized by the boundary ambiguity (Boss, 1977) created by the father's intermittent exit and return. Like many divorcing couples, Dick and Elaine found their "on-again-off-again" marital relationship continuing for several years as they resolved their ambivalence and made the transition to reorganization.

Even families that have successfully completed the earlier transitions suffer stress during this period, although they may not face severe disruption. At this time, they share their marital separation with extended family, friends, and the community as they begin the tasks of the economic and legal divorce. These mediating factors can help and/or hinder the transitional process. The family usually encounters the legal system at this time and faces additional stress in confronting the hard realities of economic hardships (i.e., splitting money, selling home) and child-focused issues of custody and care. This may also escalate the crisis, since spouses now need to divide what they had shared.

Although no-fault divorce legislation in many states reflects changing social attitudes, the legal system still requires the spouses to become adversaries, each with different attorneys. Based on a win-lose game, the legal divorce frequently escalates the spousal power struggle, adding additional stress for the family.

Transition IV: Family Reorganization

The concept of family boundaries, rules which determine the parameters of the family system (Minuchin, 1974), helps us to understand a major stress of the fourth transition, system reorganization. In the earlier transition, the absence of clear boundaries creates much of the confusion and stress; in this transition, the clarification of boundaries generates the distress. There are two major stressors with this stage: defining the coparenting relationship and deciding child custody issues.

One of the most critical and stressful tasks facing divorcing parents is that of redefining their coparental relationship, the relationship that permits them to continue their childrearing obligations and responsibilities after divorce (Bohannan, 1971). This task requires them to separate their spousal roles from their parental roles, terminating the former while redefining the latter. This complex process of ceasing to be husband and wife while still continuing to be mother and father forms the nucleus for divorced family reorganization. As Satir (1964, p. 1) has noted: "The marital relationship is the axis around which all other family relationships are formed. The mates are the 'architects' of the family." Although divorce creates structural changes in the family, the relationship between former spouses is still the key to redefinition of relationships in the divorced family.

In order for the divorcing spouses to separate their spousal and parental roles, they need to establish new rules to redefine their continued relationship. The divorced family needs to develop new structural rules which will guide their patterns of transactions (e.g., who relates to whom, when, and under what conditions?). Do the children go to mom or dad when they need money or help with school work?

In our case example, Dick and Elaine, with the help of a counselor, worked out a contract spelling out these rules and roles of their new coparenting relationship. This formal arrangement can help clarify responsibilities and, by eliminating possible disagreements, minimize conflict between ex-spouses.

These rules defining when and how each of the parents will continue to relate are critical to the child's understanding and to the stabilization of his or her relationship. Each parent needs to establish an independent relationship with the child. To do so, especially in the case of a young child, requires that former spouses continue to have some sort of relationship. How they manage and define this new relationship lays the foundation for how the divorced family will redefine itself: will it be a "single parent" or a "binuclear" family? It also determines the emotional climate or atmosphere for the process. How divorced parents define the ways in which they will share parenting can be critical to the child's psychological adjustment. Without a clear understanding of the relational rules, the child is likely to become the victim in unresolved spousal or parental conflicts. For example, if mothers and fathers continue to act out their anger with each other by fighting over visitation arrangements, the child will suffer the consequences by being upset every time he or she goes from one parent's home to the other.

Elaine and John chose a *joint custodial* arrangement, with the oldest child living primarily with his father, while the two younger children lived with their mother. Both parents continued to be involved in child-rearing tasks for all their children, however, and to share responsibility for decisions about child welfare.

Joint custody allows both parents to continue to be parents despite the divorce; proponents argue that both parents and children benefit from this arrangement (Roman & Haddad, 1978). There is some evidence that children who suffer most emotionally from divorce have been deprived of a continuing relationship with one parent. But others argue that if parents cannot get along well enough to live together, how can they share decision-making about their children? (Goldstein, Freud, & Solnit, 1973).

Transition V: Family Redefinition

The final stage of the divorce process has traditionally been the exclusion of the "problem member" from the family system. This process of "freezing out" (Farber, 1964), "closing ranks" (Hill, 1949), or "closing out" (Boss, 1977) is functional only when the father remains absent in the system. Clinical literature often cites a healthy adjustment to divorce as one when the relationships between former spouses ends (Kressel & Deutsch, 1977). The label "single parent family" as a descriptor of divorced families indicates the assumption that divorce results in one parent leaving the system (see Chapter 8).

Recent research, however, reveals that this pattern of coping with postdivorce family reorganization results in more individual stress and family dysfunction: Noncustodial fathers with infrequent postdivorce contact with their children were reported to be more depressed (Grief, 1979), more dissatisfied with their relationships with their children (Ahrons, 1980a; 1981), and more stressed regarding role loss (Keshet & Rosenthal, 1978; Mendes, 1976). Sole custody mothers were more depressed and overburdened by the responsibilities resulting from role overload (Brandwein, Brown, & Fox, 1974; Hetherington, Cox, & Cox, 1976; Weiss, 1980). Children with very limited or no father contact suffered the most severe developmental and emotional distress (Hetherington, 1979; Wallerstein & Kelly, 1980.

The nuclear family's reorganization through divorce creates new households with single parents only when one parent has no further contact with the family and no longer performs parental functions. The frequent creation of interrelated maternal and paternal households creates two nuclei which form one family system—a binuclear family system. When the family reorganizes itself as a binuclear system in which both parents continue to be part of the child's family, it helps reduce some of the distress of the divorce. The child then does not have to "lose" either parent and does not suffer such an extreme alteration of lifestyle that is so often a consequence of divorce. Parents also gain: No one parent is burdened with the single parent overload, nor is one parent forced to give up the parenting role.

The redefinition of relationships in the divorced family depends on the relationship between the parents. Although a continued, cooperative, and mutually supportive relationship between divorced parents reduces the crisis potential associated with divorce, its dynamics remain largely unexplored. The growing debate about custody rights reveals our lack of knowledge about the time-honored concept "best interests of the child" and brings the custom of sole custody into serious question. A trend toward shared custody and coparenting seems to be emerging ("One child . . . ," 1979), which should have profound implications for the postdivorce family.

Although current research on joint custody is necessarily limited to small samples, an increasing pool of data suggests a range of coparental relationship patterns which permits both parents an active role in their children's lives (Sell, 1979). One major component of the redefinitional process appears to be the parents' ability to maintain a child-centered relationship. For some this includes a personal continuing friendship, but for most it is less intimate and more task-oriented (Ahrons, 1979, 1980a, 1980b). Parents who share custody, however, experience great distress as they interact with social institutions, family, and friends. Institutions based on the nuclear family strongly resist the changes introduced by the binuclear family. For example, the request of both parents to receive copies of their children's report cards and school announcements is commonly met with resistance. Extended family and friends view such relationships as embarrassing, deviant, or in some way pathological. However, as attitudes change, social institutions will need to change in response to the needs of postdivorce families. Greeting cards are now available to announce a divorce and to send to the newly divorced. Language norms also reflect change: Phrases like "my son's mother" and "my coparent" are no longer so rare.

A family redefinition process frequently includes remarriage and the introduction of stepparents into the postdivorce family. Remarriage creates a series of transitions beyond the scope of this chapter, but which are part of the ongoing transition of family redefinition (see Chapter 9). For some families, a potential remarriage partner or spouse-equivalent may become part of the family system (one or both parents may cohabit with a significant other) prior to the legal divorce and at the early phases of the reorganization transition. Some unnamed and thus unsanctioned relationships within the binuclear family structure (e.g., the relationship between mother and stepmother) are important in the redefined family. They are kin or quasi-kin relationships (Ahrons, 1980b).

Relationships between stepparents and biological parents in the binuclear family system can provide an important emotional continuity for the child and for the whole family. It is important that a biological parent accept and respect the relationship between the child and the new spouse of his or her former spouse (e.g., that the father accept the importance of the child's relationship to the stepfather). In so doing, family redefinition is facilitated and children and parents maintain their relationships as much as possible. Without acceptance of the stepparent relationship by the biological parent of the same sex, the child is apt to suffer from severe loyalty conflicts and may have trouble establishing a good relationship with the new stepparent without feeling disloyal to the biological parent (see Chapter 9).

CONCLUSIONS AND IMPLICATIONS FOR COUNSELORS AND THERAPISTS

This chapter presents a conceptual framework for redefining divorced families and understanding the stress of divorce as part of a process of moving from a nuclear to a binuclear family. For an increasingly large segment of society, the divorced binuclear family is replacing the traditional nuclear family. Recent research suggests that the child's adjustment to divorce is correlated with his or her postdivorce family situation; a continued relationship with father and a cooperative and supportive coparental relationship are major determinants of the child's healthy adjustment.

Kressel and Deutsch (1977) define a constructive divorce as "one in which psychic injury to children is minimized, principally through the maintenance of a good coparenting relationship between former spouses." The maintenance of a good coparental relationship requires redefinition of the divorced family so that it continues to include both parents. Counselors and therapists can assist families in achieving a "constructive divorce."

Too frequently, counselors terminate their sessions with clients after helping them with their decision to divorce, or they continue to work with only one of the spouses or one part of the redefined family, the custodial mother and child. Although an interventive model is not the central purpose of this chapter, some guidelines for practice readily emerge from the conceptual framework we have presented (Ahrons & Perlmutter, 1982). The major purpose of intervention is to assist a family to redefine itself as a divorced (binuclear) family. Central to this task is the need for counselors and therapists to clarify family members' personal perceptions and values concerning divorce and to come to regard the divorced family as a continuing family system. Only then can they help the family to achieve this perception.

Major stress in divorce derives from the dramatic role transitions that are necessary correlates of family change. Divorcing spouses either lack role models or have only negative role expectations. Individuals who have had some previous exposure to a given role will adjust more easily when they are required to assume that role. To ease some of the stress of transition, therefore, counselors can provide divorcing clients with new options and access to other divorced coparents as role models through support groups for divorcing families or lectures and workshops.

Because coparenting facilitates the continuation of attachment bonds between both parents and children, some of the stress associated with loss is reduced. The redefinitional process requires helping the divorced spouses disengage from their spousal roles, at both the individual and interactive levels, while developing new rules and clarified boundaries of their continued interrelationships. With a clear understanding of the relational rules and of family boundaries, the child is then less apt to become the battlefield for spousal or parental conflicts.

Much research is needed to clarify the normative processes of divorce and postdivorce binuclear reorganization. We must better understand the processes employed by normal or healthy families so that we may identify problems in divorced families.

Finally, if we are going to provide divorcing families with routes for establishing themselves postdivorce as healthy and emotionally integrated units in society, coping strategies and rule construction processes must be made much more theoretically explicit through extensive research. Conceptualizing the process of postdivorce family reorganization is of quite a different order from perpetuating the myth of family dissolution. Systematic study, from a systems perspective, would move us considerably ahead in the development of clinical theories and intervention strategies.

CHAPTER

8

Single Parenting: Transitioning Alone

M. JANICE HOGAN, CHERYL BUEHLER, and BEATRICE ROBINSON

Most single-parent families experience a pile-up of changes and demands. Single parents must take on several roles, combining nurturing and earning responsibilities, roles which are assumed by two parents in most families. The children, depending on their developmental stage, may acquire new responsibility. Single parents may be separated, with or without legal sanction, divorced, widowed, or never-married. The family may be headed by a mother, a father, or parents may have joint custody of their children. The larger the family, the more complex the organization; children may be at different developmental stages such as preschool, adolescent, and/or adult. About 20% of all children in the U.S. live in single-parent households, almost a 50% increase since 1970. Single-parent families are most likely to be headed by separated or divorced women. About 11 million children under 18 live with their mother, and one million live with their father. Because one-parent families are a relatively small proportion of the population and deviate from the two parent norm, they experience some discrimination and/or alienation.

The number of children living with never-married mothers has tripled in the past decade, and for the first time exceeds those living in widowed families. Marital dissolution—separation or divorce—remains the major cause of single-parent families, however. Because of this, this chapter will focus primarily on divorce and separated single-parent families.

CASE STUDIES

To illustrate the nature of stress in single-parent families, three case studies follow:*

Kate Harrigan is a 30-year-old mother with children aged two and 10. She has worked in a candy factory since she was 18, taking a two-year break when her first child was born. She has been married and divorced twice, having had one child in each marriage. Although she and her second husband have been divorced for about one year, they are considering remarriage. Kate earns about $12,000 a year and receives regular child support payments from her second husband, who is actively involved in parenting their two-year-old child.

Due to the high cost of renting an apartment and the discrimination against families with children in rental units, Kate has purchased a mobile home in a suburban trailer park. Aside from housing costs, child-care expenses are a problem. She pays $250 a month for a babysitter and is unable to economize on this service. She has difficulty paying her monthly bills, especially when unexpected expenses such as car repair or special school clothes for track and Scout events are required. She has occasionally borrowed money from her second husband but has been unable to repay the loans. The cost of obtaining child-care makes it difficult for Kate to work longer hours or to spend time seeking a better job.

Reluctantly, Kate has decided to file for child support from her first husband with the aid of a relatively new law, the Uniform Reciprocal Enforcement of Support Act. This law gives every state

---

*The case studies written for this article are based on families who were involved in the single-parent project of a community-based, family counseling agency (Community Counseling Center of White Bear Lake, MN). Names and identifying information have been changed. It is important to note that many single-parent families do not seek support from public and private agencies. Therefore, these case studies may not be representative of many single-parent families.

the right to collect child support payments from a parent who is not meeting this financial obligation. Two months have passed and she has not received a check from him. Kate and the 10-year-old get into arguments about buying things, which often end in yelling, tears, and tension. Their frequent fights motivated Kate to seek help from a community counseling program for single parents.

Walter Sloan is a 45-year-old parent with custody of two adolescent sons, aged 12 and 14. His wife, Laurel, has custody of their 17-year-old daughter and their eight-year-old brain-damaged foster child. The couple is currently separated with a divorce in process.

For some time Walter had wanted a closer, more intimate and sexually active relationship with his wife. He had not considered separation until he learned that his wife had become sexually and emotionally involved with another man. The six months after he learned of her extramarital affair were the most stressful for him. At first he tried to be patient and understanding and to wait for the affair to end. When the relationship showed no signs of ending, he tried to convince his wife that they should see a marriage counselor. When she refused, he spent several months immobilized, unable to make a decision about continuing the relationship as it was or getting a divorce.

Walter agonized over his decision. He found it difficult to give up all hope that his wife might agree to work on the relationship. During the months that he struggled with the decision, he sought help from a family therapist. Walter also became very religious during those months of deciding. Once the decision to separate from his wife was made, Walter experienced tremendous feelings of relief. Walter rather quickly changed from a depressed, uncertain, and indecisive man to a more optimistic, self-assured, and motivated one. He was able to start planning for his new life with his sons. By the time the divorce was finalized, Walter was well adjusted to his new life as a single parent.

Carol Rogers is a 30-year-old parent of two preschoolers, a boy, aged three, and a girl, aged four. She dropped out of college and married at age 20. She was employed as a caterer's assistant for several years to help her husband through college. When he graduated, she quit her job and worked fulltime at homemaking and childrearing. She used her catering skills to give elaborate parties during their marriage.

One day, seemingly without any warning, her husband told her he had been having an affair with another woman and declared that he wanted a divorce. Carol was shocked, hurt, and angry. She drew on her anger to deal with the loss and grief that followed and tried to show her husband that she could be a successful single parent. She moved to a less expensive apartment and set out to find social services that could help her get started in the job world. After much searching, she discovered a government funded job training program which would enable her to finish college and enter a career. The program assisted her with child-care and educational expenses.

Carol finds it difficult to juggle the new role of single parent with that of student. The children have gotten sick on days when she has had exams and she worries that she does not spend enough time with them when major assignments are due. Since the divorce is not final, Carol worries that her husband may try to gain custody of the children. She feels that she must grant all of his sudden requests to see them, regardless of her plans. She has avoided negotiating child support and property division for fear it will trigger a custody battle.

Soon after the separation, Carol decided that she needed to have contact with single parents in situations similar to hers. She found a support group, Parents Without Partners, and regularly attends weekly events. Overall, Carol has adjusted well to the role of household head. Even her older sister, who has always been critical of Carol, has become understanding and helpful. This family support has assisted in Carol making a rapid adjustment to her new situation.

STRESSORS OF SINGLE PARENTS

As you can see from these examples of single-parent families, both personal and family concerns contribute to stress. Following divorce or death, family members may experience a sense of loss and grief. They need time to evaluate and perhaps adjust their self-images. They need to learn how they "fit" into the redefined family. With few societal guidelines or norms, ex-spouses must redefine their relationship; children often need to figure out how to relate to a custodial (i.e., parent with legal custody) and a noncustodial parent. The Sloan family, with a split custody and visitation arrangement, will need time, wisdom, skill, and patience to negotiate the rules of parent-child behavior. In the Harrigan family, child support payments continue to be an ongoing issue with Kate's first husband. Finally, in the Rogers family, child custody and property settlement are unresolved issues creating distress. Kin and community also are related to the single-parent family's ability to cope successfully, as Carol Rogers' story illustrates.

The transition to single parenting from a two-parent family begins with either informal or legal separation. The period of separation is very stressful for family members (see Chapter 7). This was true in Walter Sloan's case. In a study of spouses just before the marital separation and during the actual period of separation, Bloom and Caldwell (1981) reported that psychophysiological distress symptoms, such as headaches, rapid heartbeat, fatigue, spells of dizziness, and feeling tense, were common. Men were found to have more severe symptoms during the separation period and women reported more heightened distress symptoms just prior to the actual separation. While many of the couples who separate will eventually file for divorce, some will continue to remain separated and some will reunite with their spouses. Because of the privacy of the family, those who temporarily separate may not be known to neighbors, relatives, or census data collectors, and thus may be underreported in the literature.

Role Changes

Marital dissolution or spousal death forces both men and women to examine their family roles. Women usually face an evaluation of their wage-earning capacity, as both Carol and Kate did. Carol decided that she could not earn enough to support her family and that she would go back to college to improve her economic capacity. Kate discovered that the income from her job was not sufficient to support her family.

Traditionally, mothers have been expected to take major responsibility for child-care and other work in the home and fit their employment around family demands. Most of the fathers have "helped out" with child-care, food buying, or other homemaking tasks and have been the major wage earners. However, the phrase "help out" reveals that domestic tasks are really not part of his family job description. In a similar vein, wage earning is not an integral part of a mother's job. The father's lack of homemaking and childrearing skills and orientation, the mother's lack of a career orientation and skills, and the societal presumption that a mother is most capable of raising children are reflected in the predominance of female-headed families.

The male's lack of homemaking skills was one of the findings in Levine's (1976) study, *Who Will Raise the Children?* Evidently, the single fathers did not expect problems in coordinating the laundry, chauf-feuring, food preparation, school visits, and employment. One said, "I wasn't a full parent, (in) that I was only around in minor ways when it came to all the duties of taking care of them—arranging for doctors, dentists, and babysitters, (and) decisions if they needed new shoes." Another father who shares custody with his ex-wife reports:

> Before we split up, I spent time with the kids and I did all of the things you're supposed to do. . . . My job was to be with them at certain times, to physically be with them—to take them downtown, to read them stories—that was part of the job. . . . But now it's different (Levine, 1976, p. 39).

After interviewing single fathers, Smith and Smith (1981) concluded that those who made the transition to single parenthood most easily had "prepared" for their new roles. They had been active in both child-rearing and household management before becoming single parents. Successful role transition was experienced by those fathers who felt confident in their new role and had knowledge and resources to care for both their children and themselves.

Until recently, most men did not actively seek custody of their chil-dren. Men who did receive legal custody usually had the mother's pre-trial consent and thus did not "fight it out" in court. Within the last 10 years, however, a trend toward father-headed divorced and separated families has developed. Census data show that about 750,000 children live in these households, an increase of 184% due to divorce and 55% due to separation over the past decade. This trend may be attributed to changing beliefs about rigid sex roles and doubts about the legitimacy of presuming that mothers are always better suited to raise children. Legal scholars have argued that such a presumption may well violate the constitutional rights of fathers (Gottesman, 1981; Robinson, 1979).

The Sloan family is an example of the new trend toward father-headed families. Walter and Laurel decided to share the responsibility of raising their children; Walter has custody of their two older sons and Laurel has custody of their younger son and daughter. The way that the Sloans chose to split custody of their children reflects the traditional belief that fathers are more appropriate custodians of older male children than of female or younger children. On the other hand, the fact that Walter wanted custody of two of their children illustrates the trend toward more father-headed families.

Joint custody is another way that fathers are more actively seeking parenting responsibility for their children. Joint custody or coparenting, a relatively new legal arrangement, is aimed at maintaining a close relationship between the children and each of their parents (Grote & Weinstein, 1977). Both parents provide a home, share the child-care responsibilities, and provide economic support. Because cooperation and good communication between the coparents are essential, the courts may not recommend joint custody when there is a high level of conflict between ex-spouses. Practically speaking, parents need to live in the same community for joint custody.

Regardless of whether or not single parents choose joint custody or an informal coparenting arrangement, most single-parent families face significant role changes that create stress. Roles for family members are especially ambiguous. How are the ex-spouses going to relate to each other? What kinds of decisions about the children will be made by each parent? How will the children be involved in the decision? How much time will the children be spending with each parent? Who will be responsible for specific household tasks that the absent spouse performed? Single-parent families will need to make personal decisions and negotiate decisions with other family members in order to redefine roles.

Relatives, churches, and social groups may influence the level of stress single-parent families experience by the amount of emotional support they give to the family members as they change roles (Chiriboga, Coho, Stein, & Roberts, 1979). For example, relatives who condemn or negatively describe the single parent status of the family offer little emotional support. They may view the family as disabled, broken, and defective. On the other hand, high levels of support may be indicated by communicating acceptance of the single parent status as an alternative to the marital problems and offering child-care or other services to assist in the transition to single or coparenting. Groups such as "Parents Without Partners" and "We Care" have been organized by single-parent families to give emotional support and reduce some of the distress involved with meeting the demands of the various roles.

Parents' efforts to fulfill the provider role and other family responsibilities demand high levels of human resources. One father of a preschooler eventually gave full parenting responsibility to his parents. A mother of three children reluctantly gave up fulltime employment, stating, "I found the job rewarding but also very draining. I was attempting to take care of the kids and see friends sometimes—this plus being exhausted from the emotional upheaval—it was just too much." In the short term, employment may not relieve stress but create it. And in the long run, such nonemployment periods create irregular work histories, a major factor in low earning power.

Women who are flexible in their ideas of appropriate male and female role behavior appear better able to cope with the single-parent lifestyle. Brown and Manela (1978) found that nontraditional sex-role attitudes held by women were associated with lower distress, greater well-being, increased self-esteem, more personal growth, and a sense of personal effectiveness. This was true regardless of age, race, education, or employment status.

Economic Stressors

For many families marital separation, divorce, and spousal death create economic hardships. In the case of divorce, usually there is insufficient income to support two households. If the couple had difficulty financing the household, this change creates even greater economic disruption. Three related economic changes are common. First, income usually decreases with the loss of an adult wage earner; in the case of divorce, material goods may be divided. This change creates downward economic mobility (lower economic status) for the family. Second, the source of family income may change. Child support payments and/or government subsidies are likely to be new forms of family income. Third, families may have to temporarily or permanently change their living standards. This may include moving into low income housing or returning to the parents' household. Each of these changes will be discussed in greater detail.

Downward Economic Mobility. Overall, single-parent families have lower incomes than two-parent families. By far the lowest incomes are found in female-headed single-parent families. Table 1 shows these income differences. Female-headed single-parent families exist on about one-half of the income of two-parent familes, and about 60% of the income of male-headed single-parent families. Research indicates that few men are custodial parents and men's economic well-being after divorce often increases (Hampton, 1975). Furthermore, the literature on custodial fathers primarily addresses their child-care, day-to-day management problems, and social and emotional functioning (Gasser& Taylor, 1976; Orthner, Brown, & Ferguson, 1976; Smith & Smith, 1981).

Economic resources serve as a constraint more often for female single parents than for male single parents (Espenshade, 1979). A large number of wives and children who have never been poor begin a low income lifestyle following divorce or spousal death (Brandwein, Brown, & Fox, 1974; Duncan, 1981). While female-headed families comprise 15% of the

TABLE 1
Median Income,[a] Number of Families, and Percentage Receiving
Noncash Benefits in 1979

			Noncash Benefits			
Type of Family	Median Income	Total Number	Food Stamps	School Lunch	Subsidized Housing	Medicaid
Male-Headed Single Parent	$17,939	1,706,000	7%	7%	2%	16%
Female-Headed Single Parent	$10,300	8,540,000	29%	27%	10%	34%
Two-Parent	$21,540	48,180,000	4%	5%	1%	5%

[a]Half of the families are above the figure and half are below.
From U.S. Bureau of the Census, Current Population Reports, Series P-23, No. 110, *Characteristics of Households and Persons Receiving Noncash Benefits: 1979*, Issued March 1981, p. 11. (a)

1979 population, they account for 48% of the families living in poverty (U.S. Bureau of the Census, 1980c, pp. 41-42). Considering all female-headed families, 31% fall below the poverty level. This downward economic change includes the hardships of job discrimination against women, conflicts between employment and home responsibilities, and a reluctance by both ex-husbands and community agencies to help the female head of household. Because of the generally low incomes of single-parent families, a small cash flow (money left after necessities are paid) imposes a serious economic constraint on the management ability of the single mother. Lowered income may mean a change in buying patterns, increased debt, and a change in housing to a less expensive neighborhood.

Economic issues are pressing concerns in the two female single-parent case studies. Both Kate Harrigan and Carol Rogers developed serious financial problems following divorce. In fact, both found themselves unable to support their families with their own income. Carol obtained government aid while she went back to college to increase her earning capacity. Kate needed the child support payments from both of her ex-husbands to supplement her earnings.

Families headed by younger mothers are even more likely to live in poverty. Mothers under 25 have a poverty rate of 60%; those older have a rate of 29% (U.S. Bureau of the Census, 1980a, p. 53). Also, each additional child diminishes the woman's prospects for economic security because of the increased expenses and time required for child-care.

While parenting in single-parent families may be especially demanding, children may assist in reaching family goals. As they get older they are better able to help with the household tasks and the care of younger children. One way mothers handle the demands of working both inside and outside the home is to have the children help with the household operation (Glasser & Navarre, 1965). Children may also improve management if the single parent is trying to keep things running smoothly "for the children's sake." In this case, children serve as a motivating force for setting new goals while maintaining continuity in day-to-day living.

Changes in Source of Income. The second major economic change is the source of family income. The single-parent family may receive income from both earned and unearned sources. Wages and business investments are classified as earned income, whereas child support, alimony, public assistance, and relatives' grants are classified as unearned income. Since unearned income is characteristically more irregular and unpredictable than earned income, the ability of the family head to generate earned income is crucial.

Most single-parent families receive their main source of income from wages. In 1978, 63% of the female heads were employed; of these, eight in 10 worked fulltime (U.S. Bureau of the Census, 1980a, p. 125). On the average, females earn about a third less than their male counterparts. Reasons for this difference in wages include women's lack of job skills and experience, irregular work histories, sex discrimination in hiring practices, and limited satisfactory child-care options (Glasser & Navarre, 1965; Stein, 1970).

Several of these factors help explain Carol's and Kate's financial problems. Carol Rogers found herself unable to support her family because of her lack of job skills and experience, compounded by an irregular work history. In Kate's case, the high cost of child-care is the major reason she is unable to support her family with her salary. The difficulty in obtaining reliable high quality child-care keeps Kate from working longer hours or looking for another job.

Child support payments are low and irregular, and the nonpayment (default) rate is high. In 1978, child support was awarded to 59% of the divorced women with dependent children. Of these women, only about half received full payments, a fourth received partial payments, and another fourth received no payments at all. For those who actually received child support, the average amount was $1,800. This is a relatively small part (20%) of their total income of $8,940 (U.S. Bureau of the Census, 1980c, pp. 39-41).

Contrary to popular belief, few women are awarded alimony. In 1979, only 14% of the divorced or legally separated women were awarded payments. Of these awards, only two-thirds (69%) actually received payments and the average annual amount was only $2,350 (U.S. Bureau of the Census, 1980c, pp. 39-41). A Wisconsin study revealed that after four years 67% of the fathers had ceased paying child support and alimony (Citizens Advisory Council on the Status of Women, 1972). By this time divorced fathers may have remarried and find supporting two families difficult. A question that these parents need to reconsider is: Under what circumstances does responsibility for children end? Legally, responsibility for child support does not end with remarriage.

When spouses divorce they usually have property to divide. However, less than one-half of all divorced women have received some form of property settlement. The average settlement value received was $4,650 (U.S. Bureau of the Census, 1980c, pp. 39-41). Considering the small value of property settlements that women receive, the low and irregular child support, and infrequent alimony, it is not surprising that female-headed families experience economic stress.

When family members are not able or are unwilling to provide adequate economic support for their families, female heads may have to apply for government assistance. Public assistance includes both cash from Aid to Families with Dependent Children and other benefits, such as food stamps, public housing, school lunches, and medical care. However, only about 18% of the female-headed families receive welfare. Half of these live solely on public assistance, while the other half use payments to supplement their earnings (U.S. Bureau of Census, 1980a, p. 156).

Table 1 compares the use of government, noncash benefits by different types of families. It is clear that female-headed families use these services to a much greater extent than both male-headed single-parent families and two-parent families. This is especially true if we focus on families who use subsidized housing and medical care. Since a family must have a low income to be eligible for these services, we see additional evidence of the economic hardships faced by many female-headed families. For these families, governmental assistance may provide temporarily the needed resources to stabilize their economic situation. Carol Rogers' case illustrates this since she receives aid for college and child-care. This resource may help change her capacity to provide adequately for her family's economic needs.

The constancy of income closely relates to the parent's ability to plan expenditures, her/his sense of personal control, and self-esteem (Bould, 1977). Bould (1977) found that sources of income which are unstable and stigmatized, such as child support, alimony, and welfare, contribute to a feeling of low personal control over one's life. On the other hand, sources of income that are more socially acceptable and stable contribute to a high sense of personal control over one's life. Raschke (1977) reported that employed divorced/separated women experience less stress than those women who are dependent on others for economic support. It appears that both high self-esteem and increased personal control may help reduce stress.

The findings regarding the controlling and stigmatizing effects of accepting unearned income are clearly illustrated in Carol Rogers' feelings about accepting government financial aid in order to go to school and support her family. Carol often complained about how humiliating it was to pay for food with food stamps. In the early months of her separation, she continually fought against feelings of worthlessness and indebtedness because she needed financial assistance. After eight months and with the help of her support group, Carol was able to believe that she deserved government assistance and that she was not weak or a failure.

Changes in Standard of Living. The third area of economic change includes adjustments in family living standards. Adjustments are necessary when a family experiences downward economic mobility and a change in its source of income.

Level of living, the family's present state of well-being, is often quite different from their standard of living, their aspired state of well-being. Following divorce or separation, families may experience a reduced level of living while their standard of living remains unchanged. The discrepancy between level and standard of living will most likely generate stress. The family may need to adjust their standard of living. The adjustment process is delayed, depending on whom the family chooses as a standard of comparison. Do they use other single-parent families, two-parent families, or their own family before separation? We suggest that adjustment to the discrepancy between standard and level of living will be furthered if the family members use a realistic reference group for comparison.

COPING WITH STRESS

Management Behavior and Decision-making

It has been proposed that single-headed families can reduce some of the stress that follows divorce or death by implementing new management behavior (Buehler & Hogan, 1980). Stress-reducing managerial behavior includes: 1) setting new goals (e.g., finding a better job or returning to school); 2) adjusting the level and standard of living (e.g., having children use the bus rather than the family car); 3) exploring new resources and reorganizing routines to maximize resource effectiveness (e.g., using neighborhood food buying club to save money); and 4) redefining role expectations and negotiating task performance responsibilities (e.g., sharing housecleaning work with the children). Specific behavior may include using community resources, such as Parents Without Partners and child adult education classes for social support and to assist in formulating and reaching new goals. Children's responsibilities for household care may be increased to include a wider variety of required tasks. For example, teenagers may assume some of the shopping and chauffeuring responsibilities.

Decision-making is particularly crucial in creating new courses of action and ways of functioning (Paolucci, Hall, & Axinn, 1977). For example, Walter Sloan may decide to lower his standards for food preparation, laundry, and cleaning to encourage his sons to more fully participate in household work. Lumps in the gravy, wrinkles in the shirts, and cobwebs in the corners may be overlooked and their willingness to help praised. In Carol Rogers' case, stress prompted her to seek and weigh new alternatives for career advancement. In sum, decision-making can function to bring about desired change and thus improve family functioning.

In a study of coping strategies of divorced parents, Berman and Turk (1981) found that becoming more independent by defining a new life plan, having employment, taking care of the home, and doing more things with the children were related to positive feelings about their life. Equally important were social activities such as dating, developing new relationships and friendships, and involvement in support groups. They found that the coping strategy of expressing feelings by blowing up, crying, and getting angry was related to a low level of life satisfaction and heightened distress.

Families with high stress levels may only be able to make decisions about survival—making it through today and trying to block out decisions about tomorrow. Such decision behavior exhibits a present time orientation, defined as ongoing but not habitual behavior, what is felt and thought at the moment, and an avoidance of using a future orientation which involves more uncertainty. Future thinking requires a long-range view. While daily decisions and routines are crucial, the lack of decisions about new goals, standards, resources, and roles may limit families to a low level of functioning.

Some single parents may attempt to maintain their sex-role identity as it was during their marriage and avoid decisions that introduce much change. These "stabilizers" were identified in a study of role orientation of divorced mothers (McLanahan, Wedemeyer, & Adelberg, 1981). In contrast to those who were trying to establish a new identity, termed "changers," the stabilizers were attempting to maintain their pre-divorce roles. The stabilizers may be the single parents most likely to use survival patterns of management. Of course, at a later time, they may become changers. Survival-oriented patterns may continue as long as the single parent is committed to the same standard of living as in two-parent households. In these families, stress is generated by striving for goals and standards that are based on an unrealistic assessment of resources.

A management problem for some families is estimating the future level of available resources. For example, if Kate Harrigan decides to finance a car for three years, will she be able to make the payments? Will her ex-spouse send child support payments for their 10-year-old child? The more uncertain the parent is of child support, success in the labor market, and government services, the greater the stress. Planning ahead assumes a predictable source and amount of resources, and control over resource use.

Some families feel that they do not have the resources to reorganize—to seek and weigh alternative courses of action. In Kate Harrigan's case, the care of a young child has constrained her search for a better job; she would need to pay for child-care and take unpaid time off work. According to Janis and Mann (1977), the combined threat of continuing the present course of action and lacking time to develop better alternatives causes the stress level to remain high.

As single-parent families attempt to reduce stress, they may decide to make small changes that are perceived as low-risk alternatives. For example, Kate Harrigan may increase her hours at the factory rather than seek a job with more advancement options; she may borrow more money from her second husband to meet expenses. In contrast to developing new career goals which require comprehensive planning, Kate is surviving with small changes.

Some parents and children may pursue a goal of enlarging their social contacts. Some may adjust their level of living by eating fewer meat-centered meals. Children may assume more responsibility for helping each other. Resources may be expanded by participating in a carpool or by substituting bicycling and walking for chauffeuring activities. The evolution of change may not be readily evident in families using this incremental pattern. And since most single-parent families are faced with relatively large changes in resources and parenting tasks following divorce, making a few minor decisions may not be a very effective strategy for reducing stress.

Comprehensive management which focuses on making key, significant decisions is desirable for most families. Carol Rogers used this style of management. She moved to less expensive housing, searched for a government-supported job training program, enrolled in college, and joined Parents Without Partners. Management behavior included establishing a revised set of short- and long-range goals, deciding how childcare, household tasks, and studying would be implemented, and creating a plan so she and the children can grow and develop. Also she included day-to-day decisions involving scarce resources, such as having her sister help with the children when she has a term paper due.

Social Support

Maintaining and establishing meaningful interpersonal relations with their children and with persons outside the family is a second major coping strategy for single-parent families. For example, an important goal for Carol Rogers was to identify and utilize social support, such as Parents Without Partners and her relatives. This social network became a human resource that helped her reach educational and career goals.

Social networks, composed of relatives, friends, and/or significant others, are critical resources for single-parent families, both widowed or divorced (Brassard, 1979; Chiriboga et al., 1979; McLanahan et al., 1981; Walker, MacBride, & Vachon, 1977). As Carol Rogers stated, "I needed new friends—someone to talk to about important decisions—someone who shares the feelings of a single parent." Research on divorcing men and women found that they turned more often to informal networks to get assistance than to formal self-help groups; friends, followed by the ex-spouse, counselors, relatives, and parents, were most commonly turned to for advice and help (Chiriboga et al., 1979). Also, divorced mothers who had healthy interaction with their children have obtained support from several people within and outside the family unit (Brassard, 1979).

While in general the existence of a social network appears to be a beneficial resource, some relatives, friends and ex-spouses may create stress. According to Jauch (1977), some single parents considered in-laws supportive, whereas an equal number felt their in-laws were nonsupportive. A number of studies report that establishing a new intimate relationship reduces the single parent's stress and aids family reorganization (Hetherington, Cox, & Cox, 1976; Roman & Haddad, 1978). However, the children's perception of the new relationship will affect its contribution as a supporting resource.

Social support systems, such as the counseling center that Kate went to to help resolve the frequent fights with her children, are important too. Laws which help collect child support payments or ease estate tax burdens on widows/widowers can be of great assistance. AFDC payments, food stamps, housing assistance and private financial programs are also vital to many single-parent families, although, as discussed above, sometimes the stigma and the instability of these programs bring stress as well. Both formal and informal social supports are helpful to single-parent families' coping efforts.

In this chapter, we have reviewed the role changes and economic stressors which single-parent families face and have suggested some functional and dysfunctional ways of coping with this stress.

CONCLUSION AND IMPLICATIONS FOR COUNSELORS AND POLICYMAKERS

There are several issues that warrant the attention of families, relatives, counselors, educators, and policymakers if we are to make a society be more responsive to the growing questions of single-parent families. First is the dilemma of sex-role flexibility versus sex-role specialization. Traditionally, women are expected to take major responsibility for the nurturing role and men are expected to assume major responsibility for the earning role. Women usually fit their employment hours around family demands and later find themselves economically disadvantaged as single parents. Also, most men lack childrearing and other home-making skills and face the disadvantage of their earner role specialization in child custody arrangements. Parents and family professionals may want to examine their sex-role orientation and consider adopting an orientation that integrates earning and nurturing roles. We propose that if women had greater earning capacity and men had more nurturing skills, fewer single-parent families would be living in poverty and more divorced families would coparent their children.

Second, there is the issue of supportive networks for single-parent families. Friends and relatives can be helpful in reassuring members of the single-parent family that they are loved and cared for and not give the message that single parents and their children are part of a failure or not a "real" family. Family counselors and educators can build programs aimed at providing emotional support and information about needed services such as child-care or job training, and developing managerial skills such as goal setting, conflict mediation, and financial decision-making. If more counselors and educators could develop programs that would include comprehensive management skills, we propose that more single-parent families would improve their style of management.

Finally, public policymakers need to give attention to the guidelines for determining child custody, child support awards, and property division in marital dissolution cases. The high default rate for child support payments should be a concern of judges, lawyers, legislators, educators, counselors, and the general public. Although more study is needed, perhaps the courts should collect the child support payments in order to protect the rights of children.

More research is needed on the strengths and weaknesses of the coparenting arrangement and its effect as a cause of stress as well as a coping mechanism. Most single-parent families experience a pile-up of changes following marital separation, divorce, or death of a spouse. There are few formulas or norms for parents and children to use in making the transition from a two-parent to a single-parent family. Comprehensive management can assist families in the transition. The issues and information presented in this chapter suggest that friends, relatives, educators, counselors, and policymakers can be helpful in reducing the distress experienced by members of single-parent families.

9

Stepparenting: Blending Families

EMILY VISHER and
JOHN VISHER

Before the excitement from their wedding wore off, Tom and Sally noticed that three-year-old Michael, Sally's son from her first marriage, began asking "when was Tom going home?" Tom was unused to small children, and soon found Michael's demands for attention annoying; Tom's strong methods of discipline began to lead to arguments with Sally. And then, just when the couple was looking forward to some time alone together, Michael's father called and abruptly announced that he could not take Michael for the weekend.

Forming a stepfamily is, as this family discovered, a major role transition for every member of the family—parent, stepparent, children, ex-spouse, grandparents. Every year in the U.S. almost one-half million marriages occur where at least one partner has children from a previous marriage. As the number of divorces in this country continues to rise, so will the number of remarriages. There are already 35 million adults who are stepparents, and one child out of every five is a stepchild.

Many adults go into a remarriage expecting the impossible of themselves and of the rest of the family. Stepmothers try to be super-moms so they can overcome the "wicked stepmother" image. Stepfathers rush in and try to take command immediately, while stepchildren balk and drag their heels in resentment at being asked to participate in this new venture that has been no choice of theirs. Grandparents feel closed out and uncertain of their roles, while ex-spouses may compete for the love and loyalty of their children. Add to this crazy quilt of emotions and unrealistic expectations the ways in which stepfamilies are different from biological families, and it is clear why remarried families experience their particular tensions.

These tensions and stresses arise from the particular conditions which set stepfamilies apart from biological families: '

1) Adults and children have experienced important losses.
2) Adults and children all come with past family histories.
3) Parent-child bonds predate the new couple's relationship.
4) There is a biological parent elsewhere.
5) Children are often members of two households.
6) Family members are at different points in their individual life cycles.

These conditions mean that stepfamilies have special challenges and specific situations to which they must adapt. As in all other kinds of families, however, the method of coping with these special stressors can help the stepfamily to be a diverse, responsive, yet cohesive group.

We will consider the kinds of stresses each of these conditons generates for the stepfamily, and then consider how stepfamilies can cope with these stressors.

MAJOR SOURCES OF STRESS FOR
STEPFAMILIES

Adults and Children Have Experienced Important Losses

Remarriage with children is part of a process of family redefinition. This process begins with a death or divorce, moves to a time of single parenting, and then to a remarriage. It begins with a loss: a spouse or parent has died or there has been a divorce. There has been a tearing apart of the once-existing love relationship. Children and parents have been separated either totally or partially, depending on the custody and visitation arrangements. Sometimes brothers and sisters have been separated. There may have been a severing of relationships with grand-parents, or alienation from friends and a familiar community. And for many adults in a remarriage, many cherished dreams of marriage have been lost in the chaos of instant children and former spouses. Thus, remarriages, unlike first marriages, are born of many losses. Individuals differ in the time it takes them to mourn the losses, and frequently adults form new and meaningful relationships while children are still adjusting to a new home, a new school, new friends, or separation from a parent.

The children's view of the remarriage, then, is usually very different from the adult's view. The children's hopes and fantasies of the biological parents getting together again are dashed, and children often wonder if they will continue to see the other parent. For example, seven-year-old Kim's father was soon to be remarried. Suddenly one day Kim began to whine and demand ice cream and trips to the zoo when she was with her father. She also became cranky and disobedient during the week when she was with her mother. Kim blurted out to her mother, "Will I ever see my Daddy again?" Her expectations and fears of more loss were very clear. Parental reassurance and continued contact with her father reduced Kim's anxiety, and even though she had some difficulty sharing her father with his new wife, Kim's behavior gradually changed as she realized that she would indeed continue to be with her father as before and to have a secure place in two households.

The new couple may be happy and excited about giving the children a "full family life" again. The children, in contrast, experience new losses as they now need to share their remarried parent with another person and often other children as well. An only child may be dropped into the middle of three stepsiblings, or the favored youngest be displaced by a cute little three-year-old. A research study at the Institute for Juvenile Research in Chicago involving 41 emotionally disturbed stepchildren revealed that in 50% of these cases the symptoms began at the time of the parent's remarriage (White, 1943). Even adult children are unsure of their relation to their parents and stepparents (Visher & Visher, 1979). For "children" of any age, then, remarriage may represent loss of a close relationship with their parents, as they must now share mother or father with the new stepparent. The feelings and behavior of children at this time can cause stress for the whole family.

Adults and Children All Come with Past Family Histories

There are no identical family histories. In a first marriage the couple comes together with expectations and experiences carried from their families of origin, the families in which they grew up. Together the couple works out a unique family pattern, a combination of parenting styles, a set of traditions. Adding children to the unit is a gradual process and the babies arrive helpless and malleable, ready to assimilate the values and traditions of the family unit.

In remarriages, all individuals, children as well as adults, come together suddenly with emotional and experiential baggage in hand from their former families—their families of birth, their previous marriage families, and their single-parent households. The baggage is heavy and anything but a matched set of luggage. New roles, rules, and traditions need to be created by all these people, and everything, from the most important aspects of life to the most mundane, needs to be negotiated and implemented.

Many adults have great difficulty finding appropriate roles. Often they plunge right into the role of parents. A stepmother may try to do everything for her new family, when the children have been used to more self-sufficiency. A stepfather may try to be a firm disciplinarian, causing conflict with stepchildren and with his new wife. Our social definition of the role of the stepparent is vague at best (Fast & Cain, 1966); for example, the courts sometimes will not allow the stepparent to participate in decisions involving the stepchildren, even when it may be a change of custody involving a move into the home of that particular stepparent.

Children also wonder where they are going to fit into the new household. During the period of single parenting children have assumed new roles, and although they may have complained bitterly about cleaning the bathroom, doing the cooking, or walking the dog, they feel displaced and devalued when a stepparent or stepsiblings enter and take over these tasks. In one single-parent family, 16-year-old Laura had been doing the cooking for her father; when he remarried, the new stepmother took over the kitchen. In another single-parent household, 12-year-old Bruce had taken pride in being allowed to mow the front lawn; then suddenly, after a remarriage, the mowing was turned over to Bruce's 15-year-old stepbrother. Ten-year-old John, who had been an only child, was now expected to be a big brother to his three-year-old stepsister. As each member of the stepfamily learns his or her new role in the family and adjusts to the new roles of other family members, stress is inevitable.

Household rules and traditions which previously were taken for granted suddenly are questioned. Should children be allowed to watch television before doing their homework? How should the French toast be made? Should the Christmas tree be large or small? Live or cut? Green or white? The potential for arguments and unhappiness is obvious as these day-to-day problems are resolved.

Parent-Child Bonds Predate the New Couple's Relationship

One of the most stress-producing differences between remarried families and biological families is that in stepfamilies the parent-child relationships have preceded the new couple relationship. In first marriages couples have the opportunity to adjust to one another and form a solid couple bond before adding children to the family unit. With the birth of a baby, in the biological family each adult is a parent to the child and can influence and experience the gradual unfolding of this tiny person.

In a remarriage there is no honeymoon. The older parent-child relationships may be very strong, while the new couple relationship is a delicate and fragile union that needs the nourishment of shared, loving time together. The presence of children, uncertain of their own future in the new family, can add a dimension of turmoil that corrodes rather than enhances the new couple relationship. The couple may argue about discipline and parental roles, while children may cling to their parents for security, bang on the bedroom door whenever the adults disappear for a few minutes, and erupt with jealousy as the new group tries to forge an identity.

Many stepfamilies seem to start with the assumption that the new parent and the stepchildren will come together and love one another at once, as though they had grown up together. This unrealistic expectation can lead to deep disappointment and guilt in the family and stress for the parents and children. For example, Gwen quit her job to care for her new stepdaughter, Jenny. Gwen read to her, baked cookies for her, and tried very hard to please her. Jenny, however, pulled back as a way of coping with her own feelings of loss and loyalty to her biological mother and soon refused to talk with Gwen except when her father was around. Gwen, reacting to this rejection, became angry at Jenny and then felt guilty for her feelings. She found her husband expected her to be an instant mother to his daughter, and she did not feel she could express her emotions to him. As Gwen became more irritable, she shouted and complained more often about Jenny. In essence, a "cruel stepmother" had materialized once more, like a self-fulfilling prophecy (Visher & Visher, 1978).

Instant love is not possible because caring relationships take time to develop, and caring has much less chance to develop if there is pressure to "feel" a certain way. Anger at being told how one "ought" to feel and guilt at not loving stepchildren or stepparents not only create tension and insecurity between stepparents and stepchildren, but can also cause resentment and distance between the couple. In reaction to this demand for "instant love" between stepparent and stepchildren, parents may draw closer to their biological children. There may be anger and lack of unity between the couple; separate parent-child units within the household may eye each other suspiciously and adults with no children of their own may, like Gwen, find themselves bobbing alone on a sea of anguish. The whole situation, growing out of unrealistic expectations, can be a source of severe stress for the stepfamily.

Another situation where the pressure of parent-child bonds creates stress for the family is the situation where the stepparent's own children live with their other biological parent. A father/stepfather may feel guilty for having caused unhappiness to his children and may see his new wife and stepfamily as rivals with his biological children for his affection. He may not be able to give freely and openly to his stepchildren, but at the same time feel strong pressure to make this second family a "success." The feelings of guilt which the father/stepfather feels are often very strong; the perceived or real conflict between the parent-child bonds and the new marriage is very real and a common source of stressful emotions.

There Is a Biological Parent Elsewhere

Unlike biological families, in stepfamilies, one of the children's parents is somewhere else. Even if the parent has died, the influence of that parent remains. To love another spouse or parent often seems disloyal, memories linger and dictate present behavior, and often the new family lives in the same home, in the shadow of former friends and neighbors. One woman expressed her discomfort at living under the gaze of her husband's first wife, whose portrait, painted shortly before her death, hung in the hall of his former and her new home.

When both biological parents are alive it is difficult for parents to share children, and it is difficult for children to share parents. Many strong emotions are produced. The insecurities and pain involved in sharing children are difficult to imagine. A 32-year-old mother confided:

> My two children live with their father and his new wife. I'm married
> again to a real nice man and his job is steady but there's low pay

and I can't earn much. My kids visit every month but I worry they won't know I love them. Their Dad has lots of money. The kids know I can't give them bikes and skiis and a swimming pool, but I give them ice cream cones and trips to the zoo and swimming in the ocean and hamburgers and fries. But I keep being scared they won't love me or know how much I love them.

A sense of helplessness and lack of control colors the relationship with the ex-spouse: Reservations are made for a ski weekend, and at the last minute the children telephone to say they can't come because their mother is taking them to Disneyland; or the children are to be with their father for the weekend and the phone rings and he says he can't take them, and the mother's weekend plans are suddenly in a shambles. This helplessness to change the situation and the unpredictability of the ex-spouse's behavior can be very stressful for the stepfamily. Children, too, can feel divided between parents or households. Children might feel guilty for enjoying the company of their father, because they know of their mother's resentment and jealousy (Messinger, Walker, & Freeman, 1978).

In biological families the children may try to keep their parents' marriage together. In stepfamilies, however, the children feel a strong loyalty to the other spouse and may try consciously or unconsciously to drive the new couple apart. Loyalty to the biological parent is a very strong emotion.

Children Are Often Members of Two Households

Linked to the fact that the two biological parents no longer live together is the fact that children in many stepfamilies are members of two different households. If the adults in both households are able to work together in regard to the children, then the children go back and forth relatively easily. However, feelings of competition and insecurity are very difficult to avoid, and children may find themselves swinging between two warring camps. It may be a hot war, a cold war, or only a minor skirmish, but in each case the children are torn by their loyalty to each of their two parents.

Some children have problems dealing with "culture shock" as they go from one household to another—from American cooking to French cooking, from modern apartment to colonial home, from no TV to unlimited TV. Every household is different and there is an inevitable period of adjustment for children—and for parents—as they go back and forth.

If parents view this situation in a bitter or competitive way, then this can be a source of stress for the children and for both households.

As this summary suggests, stepfamily life by its very nature can be stressful. It should be added that the problems that other kinds of families deal with—the stresses of dual-career families or financial strains, for example, are also part of life for stepfamilies. For some of these normative stressors, however, the stepfamily setting can complicate or heighten the stressful event. For example, the stressors of adolescents in the family have been outlined in Chapter 5. But adolescents, experiencing normal conflicts about their own identity and place in the family, have a particularly difficult time in stepfamilies. The question of "Who am I and where do I fit in?" is a more acute one for them than for their younger siblings. Teenagers may be sexually attracted to stepsiblings or stepparents, and may withdraw or become hostile to mask and control these sexual feelings. They are also aware of the sexual relationship between the newly married couple. Although no systematic study has been reported, clinical observation suggests that the greatest conflict is for teenage girls faced with their mother's sexuality. Thus, normal family stressors can be complicated by the stepfamily relationships.

Family Members Are at Different Points in Their Individual Life Cycles

There are individual, marital, and family life cycles. In many biological families these cycles are congruent. In stepfamilies they often are not. For example, Ellen and Terry each started working the summer after their graduation. Six months later they married, and at the end of three years of marriage their daughter was born. Ellen and Terry were proud parents and they took great pleasure in watching their daughter grow and develop.

In contrast, Bill and Betsy had also been married for the same length of time. However, Bill was 45 and had been married before, and his 15-year-old daughter and 12-year-old son had lived with him most of the time. Betsy, 32, had not been married before. After a nine-day honeymoon Bill and Betsy moved their furniture, the children, Betsy's two cats and Bill's dog into a three-bedroom apartment. Bill's daughter spent the major portion of her time with her friends, while her younger brother stayed with his mother as much as he could. Both children "played up" to their father and excluded their stepmother.

Betsy had always dreamed of having children and longed for a child of her own. Bill, however, had risen to the top of his company and was absorbed in his work. For him having the responsibility of two children was all that he wanted.

For biological families there is an orderly progression from the marriage and honeymoon period to the birth and development of children, career advancement, the gradual separation and departure of children, on to dealing with loss as parents/grandparents die and important interpersonal relationships are cut off.

In stepfamilies there is stress because the couple may be at very different individual personal stages, the marital cycle is compressed from months to hours, and children are there from the first—often on their way to independence rather than wanting a return to family closeness—and important losses are present from the very beginning, with many partial or totally cut-off relationships.

Recognizing that there may be many clashes due to non-complementary stages can help the couple develop ways of minimizing the stress. Open discussion about having children, preferably before marriage, may prevent distress later on; setting aside time alone is important in developing the new couple relationship; realizing it will take time to feel comfortable becoming both a spouse and a parenting figure can reduce unreasonable expectations; allowing older teenagers the freedom to draw away from family and towards their peers reduces tension as they gain more independence. In other words, recognizing that there are many differing stages all competing with one another can help stepfamily members deal with the sense of confusion that can arise.

COPING WITH STRESS IN STEPFAMILIES

The methods of coping with the stresses described here vary widely, of course, with each family's situation. There are several broad strategies, however, which families have adapted to their own situations. Some of these strategies may be useful for mental health professionals in counseling stepfamilies.

Having Realistic Expectations

Stepfamilies often start off their new lives together with very unrealistic and unreasonable expectations of themselves. They believe their family must be just like a tight-knit biological family, and that every member must immediately love all the others. When, as is almost always inevitable, things do not work out quite so smoothly, stepfamily members may feel guilty, confused, and resentful. They believe their family must be abnormal or unhealthy in some way.

But stepfamilies are *not* like biological families, and loving relationships among family members take time to develop. The tension and frustration which arise out of unrealistic expectations when families try to become "normal" by forcing themselves into the nuclear family mold are a major source of stress. It does not work because stepfamilies are simply a different type of family—not better, not worse, simply different. Stepfamilies can cope more easily by recognizing these differences, accepting them, and approaching them in a realistic and positive way.

Developing these realistic expectations about stepfamily life is most important in the successful development of a stepfamily. Defining the differences in stepfamily life as sources of potential richness and reward is a very helpful attitude in managing stress. For example, families who feel strongly that children need *one* parental authority, and *one* kind of upbringing could rebel at the notion of sharing children between two households. They might worry that the children would grow up exposed to abnormal situations and be confused, comparing such an upbringing unfavorably with that of children in a nuclear family. On the other hand, families who accept these differences see the two-household life as a source of diversity. "I learned sewing and basket weaving in one home, and an appreciation of music in the other," said one grown stepchild. "I'm glad I had both homes to go to because of the rich experiences they gave me." The children have a number of adults to relate to and to use as models for their own lives. In accepting these differences, and not labeling one household as "right" and the other as "wrong," the adults as well as the children benefit from the increased diversity in their family and more easily manage what for other stepfamilies is a major source of stress.

Over and over stepfamilies confront the same myths. They are usually relieved to learn that their family can be different and still be healthy, and that family adjustment and cohesion take time—much more time than most adults expect. The deep feelings of helplessness which often accompany the ambiguity and unpredictability of dealing with former spouses are certainly difficult, but acknowledging and understanding these feelings and delineating the many areas over which family members have control will help them to cope with these feelings. For example, Joan's former husband, despite promises to change, continues to be two to three hours late picking up his children for their weekend time with him. Although Joan cannot control her ex-husband's behavior, she can see to it that the children have fun playing with friends until their father arrives, rather than insisting that they wait in the family room, bored and fuming as they listen for the sound of their father's car pulling into the driveway.

Developing New Relationships within the Family

After a death or divorce, parents often turn to their children for emotional support and together they form a very tight group. If this has happened, when the parent remarries it takes more time and thought to make a space for the new person or persons in the stepfamily group.

The situation in which Ellen found herself is illustrative. Ellen married a man, Bob, who had two children from a previous marriage. Bob felt very depressed after his divorce and had spent weekends and all vacations relating almost exclusively with his two children. The three of them enjoyed sports of all kinds and often went camping together when they had a long weekend. Bob dated only when his children were not with him.

When Bob and Ellen were married, the children and Bob continued their usual activities together and were reluctant to have Ellen join them. They felt that she did not fit in. The children wanted to continue as before, and Bob felt guilty when he suggested some other recreation or when he included Ellen in the familiar activity. There was little space for Ellen to wriggle her way into the tight family group.

In contrast, another new stepfamily planned a camping trip together. They camped in a beautiful mountain area with a lake nearby. During the weekend different groups enjoyed fishing together, playing cards together, cooking together, and hiking together. At one time the parents and children were together, at another time stepparents and stepchildren were together, sometimes the couple was alone, and at other times the entire family was doing something as a unit. In this way, new relationships were allowed to form, former relationships were preserved, and family integration began to take place.

Adults need to give themselves as well as their children the time and space they need to build trusting relationships. The couple needs to resist the inner and outer pulls on their marriage and form a cooperative unit that can be mutually supportive. Allowing time for the fragile new marital relationship to develop is very important for the stability of the whole family.

Another way of easing the transition to the new life together is to start off in a new house or apartment. Both children and adults find it easier to accept the changes in roles and in ways of doing things if it all happens in a different setting.

It is important that every family member be heard as the family negotiates new traditions and ways of doing things. Older children especially are sure of how things ought to be done, and their views need to be considered. This process of negotiation can be an opportunity for building new relationships and new traditions. The adults can share the decision-making with all family members, instead of feeling that all the responsibility rests on their shoulders. In addition, older children are much more willing to cooperate in situations in which they have had input into the decision-making process.

Understanding Children's Emotions

The feelings of adults and children may be more discrepant around the time of the remarriage than at any other time in the divorce-remarriage process. While adults are excited about the new relationship, children are resentful, hurt, and fearful. Because of this discrepancy, the adults are usually unable to fathom the children's emotions and consequent behavior. Much pain can be avoided for both the children and adults in the newly formed stepfamily if parents are aware of and sensitive to their children's concerns.

Maintaining a Courteous Relationship with the Ex-spouse

Researchers who have studied the impact of divorce on the cognitive and emotional development of children have found that the children who fare best following a divorce are those who are free to develop "full" relationships with both parents (Hetherington, Cox, & Cox, 1976; Wallerstein & Kelly, 1976; Nolan, 1977). It is important, then, that children continue to see both biological parents. The more courteous this relationship between divorced spouse and stepfamily, the more easily this sharing of children is managed and the less strain there is for all concerned.

Unfortunately, all too often the children get caught in the crossfire as ex-spouses try to hurt each other or protect themselves. Parents who are constantly angry and insulting the ex-spouse in front of the children are intensifying the split loyalties a child may feel. As one stepson said, "If Don (stepfather) and Mom say negative things about Dad, I feel I'm part of Dad to some extent, and that they're saying negative things about me." The emotional upheaval this causes for children can be stressful for the whole family. While it is important for parents to be honest about their feelings, both positive and negative, details about their negative feelings are not helpful to the children (Simon, 1964; Visher & Visher, 1979).

Adults who are divorced because they have not been able to maintain their couple relationship can still be loving parents to their children. By respecting their parenting skills and maintaining a civil contact in regards to the children, adults minimize the stress of shared parenting. Mental health professionals have come to understand that it may be important whenever possible to work with all the caretaking adults in stepfamilies to settle basic custody and visitation issues and develop more cordial relationships between adults (Visher & Visher, 1979).

Seeking Social Support

The chance to share feelings, frustrations, and triumphs with others in similar situations has proved to be an effective way of coping with many kinds of stress in families. The stresses and tensions of stepfamilies can also be eased by finding a social support network. When couples with these situations have only themselves to talk to, their tensions have less chance of dissipating and the pressures can harm and even destroy the stepfamily. Although the family may, in some cases, need special therapeutic attention, the opportunity for family members to share feelings with other stepparents, stepparent couples, and stepchildren in discussion or therapy groups, or to learn from informational materials, is proving to be extremely helpful (Mowatt, 1972; Visher & Visher, 1978). Mutual support groups and courses for stepparents are appearing throughout the United States, and organizations are forming to act as support networks for stepfamilies and to provide education for the community and for professionals who work with stepfamilies. One such organization is the Stepfamily Association of America, with the national office located in Palo Alto, California.

IMPLICATIONS FOR POLICY AND COUNSELING

The rising number of stepfamilies in the United States today suggests that schools, social service agencies, counselors, and other professionals working with children and families are seeing and will continue to see more stepfamilies. Policymakers must plan to meet the special needs of this group. How, for example, do state Aid to Families with Dependent Children (AFDC) regulations structure the child support responsibilities of the stepparent? Could schools begin to send two report cards for the child's families? Each agency dealing with families should examine its practices that may affect stepfamilies.

Social service and counseling agency administrators must assure that their staff have adequate training to be sensitive to the particular demands of stepfamilies. Specifically, therapists and counselors can help families to have *realistic expectations* about the challenges and rewards of stepfamily life. When the families realize that it takes time to build love, trust, and commitment, and that their family, though different from a nuclear family, still can be a strong one, they are often very relieved. Counselors help them anticipate the ambiguities and difficulties of stepfamily life and develop workable strategies for their family. Counselors can also help the adult members to see that the children may have different feelings about the new family than they do, and help eliminate conflict by strengthening communication among family members. Setting up local support groups for stepfamilies is also a very valuable form of assistance.

The stepfamily is a new type of American family, one which has its own stressors, challenges, and rewards. Accepting it as a good type of family and accepting its differences from other types of families can make stepfamily life more predictable, manageable, and satisfying for every member.

ENVIRONMENTAL DEMANDS ON THE FAMILY

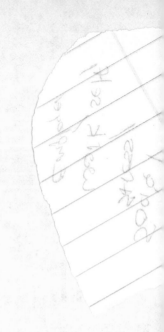

CHAPTER

10

Family Adaptation to Environmental Demands

GAIL F. MELSON

Amanda Jones is jolted rudely awake from sleep by stereo noise from the apartment below. It is 2 p.m., time to get ready for the 3-11 p.m. shift at the hospital. Sam, Amanda's husband, should be home at 6 p.m. from his shift at the plant. The kids manage pretty well for themselves after school until Sam gets back, Amanda reassures herself, but the older (14-year-old) boy is getting hard to keep track of. The trouble-making crowd he's hanging out with is worrying Amanda, who has other things on her mind—how they're going to pay for fixing Mary's teeth, rumors of more layoffs at the plant, just getting from payday to payday. And work. Sure, I'm grateful to have it, Amanda thinks, but if they get any shorter on staff at the hospital, they'll be asking the patients to get up and take care of themselves. Amanda doesn't like to think of the ride home on the subway. Even with escort service to the station, even traveling in a group, she's terrified until she hears the locks on her door thud into place, sounds that say, "You're safely home again."

A hundred miles away, in a small farming community, Amanda's country cousin, Alice, is driving from the store where she works as a

clerk to what she bitterly describes as "the family homestead." The
trailer, temporary shelter until they build their home next to
George's father's place, has been their house almost seven years now,
and moving out seems more and more remote, despite the three little
kids. We live just like a bunch of sardines, she mutters. Time was,
we were going to be a real *farming family, just like George's*
parents. Some *farming family, she thinks, me at the store, George*
picking up construction, odd jobs, working a section for his father.
Hardly an acre of our own, really. And each year, Alice realizes,
George seems to get quieter, turning in on himself, only to explode
suddenly in one of his rages. "If this keeps on," she suddenly says
aloud, "I'm leaving, I swear I will."

Amanda and Alice, mythical city and country cousins, are experiencing much of the environmental stress felt by many American families, stress related to economic hardship, employment conditions, and urban or rural living. These and other issues are explored in other chapters in this section. The goal of this chapter is to present a framework for understanding such questions as: What is environmental stress? Why do individuals and families differ in their perception of and ways of dealing with stress? What are the most important sources of stress from the environment outside the family? How can families better cope with environmental stress? Is all stress detrimental? If not, what levels of stress are optimal? This framework, called an *ecosystem* model, will consist of interrelated concepts to help define stressors, assess their impact, and describe mechanisms for changing overly stressful situations.

A FRAMEWORK—THE ECOSYSTEM MODEL OF ENVIRONMENTAL STRESS AND THE FAMILY

Because the term *environment* is so widely used in so many different ways, misunderstandings have developed about what precisely it means.

Strictly speaking, the environment of a family is anything outside of that particular family. However, the word environment has been used to refer to different aspects of the world outside of the family unit. For example, one might mean the *immediate physical setting* in which the family is located, the dwelling which the family inhabits, the school building to which the children go each day, the office, factory, store, hospital or other workplace, the college library where you may now be reading these words.

Such specific places where individuals and family units engage in specific activities as part of their roles, usually during specified times, have been termed *microsystems* (Bronfenbrenner, 1976) or *behavior settings* (Barker, 1968); but whatever the term, the focus of interest is on the *immediate physical context* in which family members come face-to-face with each other and with other people.

In the life of any family member, multiple microsystems are involved. Like our fictitious Alice, we waken in one microsystem, usually work in another, spend time in transit to yet a third, meet friends in still other settings, and so on. Taken together, all the microsystems which regularly involve an individual have been called the mesosystem of that person (Bronfenbrenner, 1976). Individuals (and families) vary in the number of different microsystems in which they participate, as well as in the ease or difficulty with which transitions from one to another can be made. We may contrast the person who works at home, with neighbors for friends, with another who changes microsystems from work to leisure to family. As daily commuter traffic jams attest, such changes are often time-consuming moves from geographically distant microsystems. As we later discuss how environmental characteristics contribute to stress in families, we will be referring to the role played by the number of microsystems and the cost of making transitions among them.

The collective microsystems of the individual, or the mesosystem, will also differ in the degree of congruence or contradiction in demands made on the individual. Microsystems, or behavior settings, have demands, usually unstated, for proper behavior. For example, it is proper to jump up and down and scream in the microsystem of a college basketball game, but improper to engage in the same behavior in a college lecture hall. At work as a department store clerk, Alice is expected to show a smooth, impersonal, but pleasant style of relating to people, one she must put aside in the microsystem of her home, where intimate, genuine emotions with family members are necessary.

We shall see that stress may also be understood in terms of the nature of the different demands made on family members as they move from one microsystem to another.

While each family member has her own mesosystem, one can compare the mesosystems of each family and ask: How similar are these mesosystems? In other words, how many settings do family members share in common? How often are they likely to encounter one another in these settings? For example, Amanda and her husband Sam share the same home, but because of different work shifts, they are in that home together only for a few hours late at night. Their children interact with both parents there only during weekends. By comparing the mesosystems of each family member, we can see how the environment can either encourage or discourage shared experiences.

Thus far, we have been considering the term *environment* to mean concrete, immediate physical settings only. Yet *environment* is also used in a more global, less easily observed sense. Influencing how individuals function in their microsystems in the exosystem, a term used by Bronfenbrenner (1980) to refer to the actions of major institutions operating on the local level, including the neighborhood, work world, mass media, government agencies, and transportation facilities. Finally, on a still more global level, the macrosystem (Bronfenbrenner, 1980) may be defined as the overarching institutions of the culture, such as its religious life, political system, or economic organization. This larger culture gives meaning and character to daily life as enacted at the microsystem level.

Thus, each aspect of the environment we have defined moves from specific to more inclusive. *Each dimension of the environment influences the others.* For example, the educational system of a society (macrosystem) affects the organization of the community schools (exosystem), which in turn affects a specific child in a specific school (microsystem). What goes on in this school will be felt in the other microsystems, such as the home. If a child is defined as a behavior problem at school, he may begin to fight with his siblings, or, just as likely, may exhibit conspicuously model behavior at home, as if to say, "The trouble is in that setting, not in me."

In summary, we may think of environment as a widening circle of influence, from the immediate physical setting to the cultural context.

ENVIRONMENTAL SOURCES OF STRESS

Environmental Demands and Fit

We are ready to describe a framework for understanding when and how environmental events are stressful to families. To do so, we must first introduce two other concepts—demands and fit.

It is useful to think of families (and the individuals within them) as having demands which they make upon the environments in which they find themselves. These demands are expectations (usually unspoken), about what the environment ought to provide. What are such demands? At the very least, families demand an environment that allows them to maintain some minimal sense of identification as a family unit. Beyond that, each family will differ in its demands for emotional closeness, communication, flexibility, and solidarity. They will need an environment which makes possible their image of family life. So, too, families will differ in the amount of stimulation, change, and stability in the environment that they find optimal.

Just as families differ in their demands, so do environments differ in the demands they make upon those functioning within them. As we pointed out earlier, some family members move in and out of many microsystems during a typical day, while others experience fewer settings. Thus, for any family member, the *number of microsystems* and the ease of making *transitions* among them may be thought of as environmental demands. Secondly, any single microsystem may be thought of as having its own set of expectations for behavior, or demands. There may be many such demands, or the setting may be a relatively "hang loose" one, in which a wide range of behavior is tolerated. For example, some workplaces have specific expectations for employee dress, language, and social relations in addition to rules about work performance. Not only do microsystems differ in total number of demands, but they also differ in the complexity and coherence of these demands. We may ask: How difficult to fulfill are the demands of a microsystem? Are these demands contradictory, so that, for example, people in this setting are expected to be both aloof and intimate?

Complexity and contradiction may exist, not only within a single microsystem but at the mesosystem level. Thus, one setting in which the individual functions may demand a certain set of behaviors, while another setting requires very different behaviors. Particularly in modern industrialized societies, people are accustomed to moving in and out of widely different contexts. The urban worker may wake in the morning, ride a packed subway, work in an office with a small group, eat lunch alone, drop in later at a party, jog in a nearly deserted park. Such a day is composed of many worlds, each differing in "appropriate" stimulation level. A subway car with 50 people seems almost empty, but the same 50 people on the jogging path create an intolerable crowd.

Each microsystem is characterized by a particular level of change and stimulation. Environments with high levels of stimulation require abilities quite different from less stimulating settings. Environments whose levels of stimulation change rapidly demand greater flexibility than relatively unchanging surroundings. Finally, environments containing contradictory, ambiguous information demand skills that go untested in a simpler setting.

Thus far, we have been considering environmental demands on the individual. But when the family is considered the unit of analysis, we become interested in the *total number of microsystems* involving the family, as well as the degree of *overlap* in microsystems among family members (e.g., the relationship between the demands made in the microsystems of the father and those made in the microsystems of the mother). If little overlap in microsystems exists, individual schedules may be pulling family members physically apart. The nature of environmental demands made on such a family will be quite different from those made on family members who spend significantly more time together.

Demands also exist at the exosystem and macrosystem levels of the environment. Through numerous regulations and informal expectations, individuals experience the changing policy directions of school systems, work world, political institutions, and mass media. Thus, schools may emphasize individualized explorations of knowledge in open classrooms or the acquisition of basic skills by the whole group in more structured classrooms. During periods of rapid social change, exosystem demands may be felt as ambiguous, contradictory, and unpredictable.

At the macrosystem level, where environmental demands stem from the overarching institutions of a culture, it is clear that cultures differ in the number, complexity, ambiguity, and rate of change of their demands. For one thing, cultures differ in values and behaviors defined as adaptive. One society may emphasize respect for one's elders, reverence for tradition, and family solidarity, while another may stress independent achievement and orientation towards the future. Cultures also differ in the rate at which they are experiencing change. In Third World countries undergoing rapid technological development, the worlds of tradition and Westernized modernity coexist and intermingle, making for a complex set of demands. There people may work in high-rise office buildings in the city, while at the same time maintaining close ties to their traditional villages.

Stressful situations may be defined as ones in which individuals or families recognize a poor *fit* between their demands and those of the environment. Because of such a discrepancy in demands, the normal range of functioning is inadequate to satisfy needs and expectations. What is defined as a stressor (or stressors), the source of the stressful situation, will depend upon how the person or family interprets this situation of discrepancy in demands. Does the problem lie in the demands made on the environment by the individual or family or by the environment on the person? Or both?

For example, a family that needs to spend much time together will experience stress if little overlap in individual mesosystems exists. Individual schedules pull family members in different directions, so little time is available to spend together. Because the demands of family and environment conflict and the normal functioning of the family does not resolve this conflict, stress is experienced. Is the stressor the family's need to be together, or is it the separate microsystem involvements of family members? Note that the stress itself is defined in terms of the interaction between people and their settings. However, indentification of the stressors depends on how the family understands its situation.

Although we can think of stress felt by either individuals or family units in terms of these concepts of *demands* and *fit*, understanding *family* stress is considerably more complex than thinking about individual stress, since the family represents a multiplicity of individual demands, perceptions of the environment, and understandings about the sources of stress. Individual differences in personal history, temperament, and attitudes make it inevitable that differences will exist within families—not just between families—in the perception of environmental demands, person demands, and hence, the degree of fit between the two.

Adaptation and Change

Just as we have characterized stress in terms of lack of fit between environmental and family demands, we can define adaptation of family to environments as "good fit." One must not conlude that stress or lack of fit between family and environmental demands is "bad" and that adaptation is, therefore, "good." The question of values is a separate one. Families can adapt to conditions that are physiologically and psychologically harmful to them. They can respond to adverse environments by developing destructive, abusive interaction patterns. Such patterns may fit environmental conditions very well, becoming stable and even resistant to change. Adaptation does not necessarily denote a "successful" individual or family, just as stress is not necessarily a condition from which families flee.

Since the demands of families and of environments are constantly changing, one must consider the concepts of stress and of adaptation as dynamic ones. Families and the individuals within them change in the demands they make, not only on one another but also on the environment outside the family. Returning to our profiles of Amanda and Alice, we see many ways in which family demands change over time. When Alice and George first married, their trailer was viewed as an adequate family dwelling, but after seven years and three children, their demands had changed. Similarly, the work arrangements of Amanda and Sam, which leave the children unsupervised after school, are becoming increasingly worrisome as their children join adolescent peer groups.

These are examples of changes in family demands in response to changes within the family. New family members are added, while individuals within the family change. Families may also change the demands they make of the environment because their values and expectations may change. The more information families acquire about the range of possibilities open to them, the more they may be expected to revise their expectations. Hence, increased education may lead to greater dissatisfaction about aspects of family life and greater willingness to work for change.

Changes in environmental demands also occur. Within any microsystem, such as a work setting, individuals are subject to changes in workshifts, layoffs, plant openings, new regulations, and relocations. In the school microsystem, school closings, teacher changes, school population shifts, and moves from one school to another are evidence of changing environmental demands. No matter what microsystem we consider, environmental change is the rule, not the exception. Such change may occur in the nature of the demands made (e.g., when new regulations are introduced), in an increase or decrease in the total number of demands (e.g., when a teacher announces he will no longer take attendance), or in an increase or decrease in the ambiguity or contradictoriness of demands themselves (e.g., when the boss's remarks about employees' appearance seem to be suggesting a dress code, but no one is sure).

Changes in environmental demands occur not only within a single microsystem, but in the relations among microsystems, or the *mesosystem*. When a plant relocates to the suburbs, this may make it difficult for some employees to make the daily transitions from home to work to day-care center. Here, environmental demand has increased the cost of moving from one microsystem to another. Demand may also change in the degree to which the different microsystems of an individual are congruous. An example might be when conditions at work change so suddenly that work and family commitments conflict. Such changes in environmental demands are felt not only by individuals, but also by family units.

Rapid Social and Technological Changes: Future Shock. Macrosystems, or cultures, differ in their rate of change. Contemporary American society has been characterized as one in which environmental change is very rapid. Alvin Toffler's bestseller *Future Shock* (1970) drew popular attention to the effects of accelerated rates of change in technological innovations, in information gathering, and in general lifestyles. Toffler argued that such rapid change created mass susceptibility to the condition of "future shock," defined as "the distress, both physical and psychological, that arises from an overload of the human organism's physical adaptive systems and its decision-making powers" (p. 326).

Future shock arose, Toffler stated, because of inherent limitation in the ability of humans to process new information. Accelerated change presents more information to people than they can make available for intelligent choice. Toffler did not see environmental change itself as a problem. Rather, he emphasized the importance of an optimal rate of change, the limits of adaptation, and the physical and psychological toll that highly accelerated change can exact.

The effect of an accelerated rate of change on the family has become the subject of considerable debate. In an age of impermanence, perhaps the family becomes more important than ever as a haven from the turbulence outside. As other relationships are made and broken easily, increasing burdens are placed on the family to fulfill needs for acceptance, permanence, and trust.

Others argue that the family is just as vulnerable as any other institution to effects of change. For example, in a "future-shocked" society, parents would be unable to predict their children's future life as adults; hence, they would be unsure about what values, skills, and behaviors would be most important to teach them.

While some aspects of contemporary life fit Toffler's picture of the future-shocked society, it is perhaps overdrawn as a severe challenge to family adaptive capacities. For one thing, many Americans stay put, value roots, and enjoy stable family networks and predictable community surroundings. Moreover, even in situations of rapid change, there are certain strengths within families that may cushion adverse effects. Studies of family functioning during periods of social upheaval sometimes find the family remarkably resistant to disruption. Not only does the family have built-in sources of stability in the face of change, but it may be the one institution in society that can absorb and respond to changes effectively. Vincent (1966) has emphasized the *adaptive function* of family. The family responds to changes both externally and from within. It also contributes to change in the larger society, or macrosystem, by socializing children to take on new roles. Vincent emphasizes not how the family is buffeted by societal changes, as Toffler does, but how the family is the agent promoting orderly change in the society.

To recapitulate, we have defined stress in terms of lack of fit between environmental and family demands, emphasizing the changing nature of both environment and family.

COPING WITH ENVIRONMENTAL STRESS

Families make many different kinds of responses in order to achieve better fit between environmental and family demands. For example, Alice can respond to the crowded conditions in their trailer by blaming her husband, by denying that any problem exists, or by leaving the family entirely. She may become overwhelmed with anger at the whole situation, unable to separate in her mind those elements that can be changed from those elements that cannot. She may search actively with her husband for alternatives or remain rigidly closed off to new information. Those actions which make it possible for the family to understand, shape, and master the environment, as well as themselves, have been called *coping responses* (Haan, 1977). Such actions help the family recover from the disruptive effects of stress and allow them to reorganize. However, coping, in promoting better fit between environmental and family demands, does not necessarily remove conflict or return the family to the status quo.

Family Characteristics and Family Functioning

Many factors influence a family's coping behavior. Family *characteristics* are important. The resources afforded by higher income and education often enable the family to achieve better fit between environmental and family demands. With more money, Amanda could hire someone to supervise her children while she and her husband worked, and Alice could move to more spacious quarters. With increasing education comes more knowledge about alternatives.

However, the distinctions of class, income, and occupation do not always enable us to predict the coping patterns of a family under stress. Aspects of family functioning are also important. Families competent at meeting crises have been found to have a nonmaterialistic value orientation, to perceive emotional problems as appropriate family concerns, to identify accurately family problems, and to share decision-making powers among family members. Competent families have been found to be cohesive, open to communication from within and outside the family, and capable of dealing with tensions, rather than tension-free (Hansen & Hill, 1964; Hill, 1965). Other studies have found competent family members to expect that most of their encounters with people will be positive experiences, and to respect the views and feelings of others. They demonstrate initiative and energy in responding to problems (Lewis, Beavers, Gossett, & Phillips, 1976).

Children's Coping

Families also differ in the extent to which they promote the development of coping skills in children. Research has found (Baumrind, 1967; Haan, 1977) that children who are good copers tend to have parents who are warm, loving, supportive, conscientious, and good at communicating. While respecting their child's independence, these parents hold firm to their convictions about what is right, explaining their reasons to the child, yet insisting on proper behavior. This *authoritative* style of childrearing has been contrasted to both the *authoritarian* (controlling without warmth) and to the *permissive* (noncontrolling but warm) styles.

It is important to note that this research does not show that certain parenting styles *cause* coping skills to develop in children. The association found between parenting styles and children's coping can also be explained as a parental response to an already skilled coper. It is easier to be warm and to enforce clear standards with a child who is friendly, competent, and self-reliant than with one who is hostile, passive, and incompetent. Of course, the original source of the child's competence is still a question which needs to be answered.

Not only do families differ at any one time in the characteristics which promote coping with stress, but also, over time, particular periods in the life of any family may be particularly difficult (Rodgers, 1973). These are times when environmental demands may be high just when family coping resources are low. For many families, the early childrearing period is just such a time. New financial obligations are undertaken just when income may drop because the wife may have recently left employment. Thus, it is not surprising that families with young children report more dissatisfaction with jobs, level of living, and the financial cost of children than families with adolescents or older children.

Social Support

The sources of coping lie not only within the family but also outside it. Familes do not exist in isolation. First, the family has kin and quasi-kin relations that can cushion it against stress. For example, the adaptation of Appalachian migrants to an urban-industrial work situation was studied (Schwarzweller & Crowe, 1969). The investigators found that those migrant families who were able to use the wider family support system were better able to cope with the many changes in their lives. Frequent, intense, and useful interactions with relatives has been termed *extended familism* (Winch & Greer, 1968). Relatives can take over family functions such as child-care, share material resources through loans and gifts, and provide information and contacts the family may need. Friends, neighbors, and coreligionists may also be part of support groups. For example, many European immigrants to this country were aided by "home town associations," comprised of individuals coming from the same area of Europe. These associations provided financial and other assistance.

Changing Environmental Demands

Coping is affected not only by family characteristics, but also by environmental characteristics. After all, the lack of fit between environmental and family demands may be narrowed by changing environmental demands, rather than changing the family. If work schedules do not permit children to be supervised, one solution is to change such schedules to build in greater flexibility for parents. Such flextime arrangements have been successfully instituted in some enterprises. Similarly, business can take family needs into account in planning employee relocation, workshifts, or executive responsibilities. Similarly, if families feel that schools are unresponsive to their children's needs, they may focus on changing the child to better fit the school, or work to make the school more responsive to the child (or both).

Families use two broad strategies for changing environmental demands to achieve a better fit (Melson, 1980). Stimulus regulation involves family efforts to selectively "let in, delay or shut out" demands to minimize family disruption and exhaustion of its resources. Stimulus regulation also involves setting priorities on those things which demand time—the Boy Scouts vs. soccer team, or taking a night class vs. an evening out with friends. Environmental control, another process of family adaptation to lack of fit, refers to the important component of self-direction in processing stimulation. One author (Mechanic, 1974) has suggested that people approach the environment with *plans*, seeking information, shielding themselves from unwanted stimulation, and keeping options open for future changes in direction.

Specifically, families can seek to change environmental demands by addressing the following sources of lack of fit: reducing (or increasing) the number of microsystems involving family members, working for greater clarity of demands with an "ambiguous" microsystem, agitating for greater sensitivity of one microsystem to the demands of other microsystems involving the family, and working to provide facilities that will make transitions among microsystems easier and less expensive.

Coping through environmental change requires concerted group efforts aimed at making an impact on the environment. Individual families in isolation can do little to reduce pollution, provide better health care and child-care services, or make education more relevant to their needs. The ability to organize and press for demands is as much a family coping skill as authoritative childrearing or open communication.

CONCLUSION

In summary, we have presented a view of stress as lack of fit between family and environmental demands. In so doing, the emphasis has been on the importance of defining stress relative to family perceptions and needs and, most important, relative to the interaction of family with environmental settings. We have used Bronfenbrenner's concept of a nested series of interlocking environments—microsystem, mesosystem, exosystem, macrosystem—to show how families make demands of these environments and how these environments, in turn, make demands of families. Family adaptation has been depicted as efforts at maintaining a relatively good fit between these two sources of demands. Coping is defined as those active efforts which allow the family some mastery over its environment. Given the fact of nearly constant change in both family demands and environmental demands, the family is in a dynamic, reciprocal relationship to its environments.

The four chapters in this section illuminate some specific kinds of environmental stress—whether it be balancing demands of work and family microsystems, dealing with stressors from social or physical environment, as Black or rural families must do, or managing the financial pressures of inflation.

11

Work and Family: Achieving a Balance

JOYCE PORTNER

Meisha is 27, works in a factory, and is a single parent. She finds her days exhausting. Her shift starts at 7:00 a.m., so she must be up by 5:30. She leaves her two sons, ages 12 and 9, to sleep a bit later, but calls to wake them when she gets to work. Once in a while she'll get a call from them about some minor emergency, but even when they don't call, she worries about how they're doing. While her supervisor at work understands her dilemma, he is very concerned about her performance on the job.

Brett, 40, works for the same company, but is a senior manager. He has a much more flexible job than Meisha, with an excellent salary, and lots of perks and benefits she does not have. But the job demands for him are also serious, with a regular 60- or 70-hour workweek. In addition, his wife, Erin, has a career of her own, and is unable to fulfull the traditional supportive role of the corporate wife. Because both Brett and Erin have demanding jobs they are attuned to what their partner's job pressure means. Their high level of income allows them to hire both household help and child care. However, Brett is concerned about how they are raising their eight-year-old son; is he

*getting enough of their attention? There just never seems to be
enough time.*

These two situations show the wide range of American families attempting to balance the sometimes competing demands of work and
family life.

Over the past decade, increasing attention has been paid to these
demands: Conferences, magazine articles, television specials, and coffee
break conversations have all highlighted work/family stressors and the
search for solutions that more and more families are struggling with.
This search is likely to gain more momentum.

The necessity for juggling of work and family roles has, in part, been
created by the dramatic changes that have taken place in American
families in the last 20 years. In the 1950s, 70% of all households were
made up of a working father, a homemaker mother, and one or more
children. Today, only 15% of American housholds have this family form
(Yankelovich, 1981). This change is due to the fact that there are more
women working outside the home, more child-free couples, and more
single parents and single-person households. In particular, the increase
in dual-earner and single-parent housholds generates the potential for
great work and family stress.

One research study has found that more than a third of all workers
who are married or living with a child under 18 experience significant
work/family stress (Pleck, Staines, & Lang, 1980). As might be expected,
working parents, particularly those with preschoolers, reported more
stress. The family members participating in this study identified three
major conditions creating work/family conflict: excessive work time,
schedule conflicts, and fatigue and irritability brought home from work.
Husbands were more likely than wives to report excessive work time
as the major cause of work/family conflict, while wives were more likely
to report fatigue and irritability. Female single parents were more likely
to report schedule incompatibility as the major problem.

Work/family stress is experienced differently by families depending
on how they allocate employment roles and household roles. In two-
parent families, two major patterns exist, each with a subpattern (Portner, 1978). In the traditional breadwinner/housewife pattern, the husband performs all of the employment functions and the wife virtually
all of the household work functions. In the dual-employment pattern,
husband and wife are each responsible for employment and household
responsibilities. In 1978, 51% of all married couples were dual-employment couples and 33% were traditional couples. The remainder had no
earners or the husband was not an earner (Hayghe, 1981).

The subset of the dual-employment pattern is the dual-career pattern which was discussed in detail in Chapter 6. In this pattern, both husband and wife have careers which require time and energy obligations beyond work time, and both place a high emphasis on advancement. The career situation usually requires extensive preparation, education, and a high commitment to the profession, not just the employer. Approximately 14% of dual-employed couples can be classified as dual-career couples (Hayghe, 1981).

The subset of the traditional pattern is the two-person single-career pattern (Papanek, 1973). In this pattern, the wife has implicitly expected social and home responsibilities (such as business entertaining, community volunteer work, child-care, home maintenance) that are particularly designed to free the husband's time for more intense work involvement. The two-person single career is often found in corporations, law, ministry, politics, and academe.

In single-parent families, the employment roles/functions and household roles/functions are fulfilled entirely by one person, almost invariably a woman. About 15% of American families are headed by women (General Mills American Family Report, 1981). Lack of a spousal "back-up person" for employment and household responsibilities creates even greater work/family stress, as was discussed in Chapter 8.

In families where the adolescents are employed, it is not uncommon for three or four family members to be confronted with work demands as well as family responsibilities.

Some work/family stressors cut across all these patterns, while others are unique to a specific pattern. This chapter focuses first on stressors common to these patterns, although generally experienced somewhat differently by each type of family. Coping strategies and resources for combating these work/family stresses will be presented; some of these are attitudes and skills of the family members and others are assistance which is provided by the employer or community.

WORK/FAMILY STRESSORS

Work/family stressors are issues which must be resolved by family members in order to have a satisfying balance between work and family life. In this chapter, the focus will be on chronic stressors such as long work hours, take-home work and take-home worries, child-care arrangements, and allocation of household responsibilities. A very common work/family stressor, unemployment, is discussed in Volume II of *Stress and the Family*.

Significant sources of work-related stress for families include the attitudes or expectations family members and others have regarding work/family role performance, and the allocation of time and energy regarding family roles. It is important to note that not all families perceive all problematic work/family issues as negatively stressful. Stress may be perceived as stimulating or energizing, and a life without stress seen as boring or purposeless. Stress can serve to clarify objectives and to increase creativity, problem-solving ability, cohesiveness, and emotional involvement.

Expectations as a Source of Stress

The way we perform our work and family roles and the satisfaction we feel about these roles are shaped by various kinds of expectations we or others have about these roles. Some expectations are related to social norms or ideals about what mothers or fathers ought to do. Other expectations are those we have of ourselves. Still others are expectations our employers have of us.

Perceived Social Expectations

Both men and women perceive definite social expectations regarding work and family roles. Columnist Ellen Goodman poignantly illustrated a dilemma faced by many women (Goodman, 1981). A student in one of her classes asked with an angry undertone, "Why is it that working women always act as if women at home were somehow inferior?" This was juxtaposed with the question of another student, "Why do women at home always act as if women who go to work are bad mothers?" No matter which route is taken, many women feel defensive—attacked and denigrated by much of society.

Goodman's resolution of the issue was: "The toughest question is, finally, the one I was never asked: Why is it always so difficult for any of us to simply say: 'I am choosing this way, not because it's right or wrong, but because, on the whole, it seems best for me . . . for mine . . . for now'?"

Women who choose to work outside the home and women who choose not to both feel equally attacked by society today, partly because of the equal split between employed and non-employed American women. Fifty-one percent of all women are employed (Fullerton, 1980) and 49.4% of married women are employed (Johnson, 1980). When half the members of a group do something, a "societal tipping point" is reached (Bernard, 1975, p. 75). Normlessness results from such a 50-50 balance—there is no "definitive consensually accepted norm." Consequently, the woman feeling ambivalent about her choice may well perceive herself to be attacked. Rather than falling unthinkingly into a proscribed work/family pattern, women today must consciously evaluate their position and make hard decisions.

Similar dilemmas are beginning to be experienced by some men as they question the price of occupational success or the extent to which they wish to be involved in parenting. Both men and women may find that they occasionally reevaluate the balance in time and energy they devote to their work and family roles. Major transitions requiring readjustments in time and energy, either at home or at work, are likely to reactivate questioning about societal expectations. For example, the woman who has chosen to work and feels strongly committed to this decision may be surprised when she finds herself questioning this course of action with the birth of her first child. A man, offered a promotion involving greater work time and travel, may unexpectedly be torn about accepting it because of the repercussions of this decision for his family.

When a couple freely chooses the work/family pattern they want, there are benefits for the marriage, for children's personal adjustment, and for mother-child relationships. Marital satisfaction, development of children's attitudes and abilities, and adequacy of mothering are likely to be more positive for a couple that has voluntarily chosen a work/family pattern, whether that be the dual-employment or the traditional pattern (Hoffman, 1974; Orden & Bradburn, 1969).

Intermittent employment may also be used to cope with these demands. A parent may stop working for a time, typically when the children are young, and then reenter the labor force when family responsibilities lessen. Or a parent may psychologically retreat by reducing commitment to the occupation in favor of expanding involvement in the family sphere. This may involve change in work responsibilities or lessening of work time. Reentry occurs as the children grow more self-reliant.

Self-Expectations

At times, the expectations we have of ourselves regarding work and/or family roles create additional stress. Two of the dysfunctional syndromes that occur are superwoman/superman patterns and workaholism.

A "superperson" is one who expects to manage a career, home, and family with complete ease, expecting to maintain a perfect job, a perfect

marriage, a perfect house, and perfect control of children. Family scholars have found the work/family stress is greatest when the work role
and the family role are perceived as equally important (Gilbert, Holahan,
& Manning, 1981).

Ellen Goodman humorously portrays the plight of the superwoman:

> Super Woman gets up in the morning and wakes her 2.6 children.
> She then goes downstairs and feeds them a Grade A nutritional
> breakfast and then goes upstairs and gets dressed in her Anne
> Klein suit and goes off to her $35,000 a year job doing work which
> is creative and socially useful. Then she comes home after work
> and spends a meaningful hour with her children because, after all,
> it's not the quantity of time—it's the quality of time. Following that
> she goes into the kitchen and creates a Julia Child 60-minute gour-
> met recipe, having a wonderful family discussion about the checks
> and balances of the U.S. government system. The children go up-
> stairs to bed and she and her husband spend another hour in their
> own meaningful relationship at which point they go upstairs and
> she is multi-orgasmic until midnight (Goodman, 1979).

The reverse of the superperson who wishes to excel in all roles is the
workaholic, who pours all attention into one role—the job. The workaholic's work life is so central that it severely and chronically interferes
with family and personal life. Although the workaholic may enjoy and
be addicted to this pattern, it is usually the family and work colleagues
who suffer from the excessive drive and dedication to work (Machlowitz,
1980).

The term "corporate bigamy" was coined to describe workaholics who
are seemingly married to their job as well as to their human mate (Feinberg, 1980). One author's opinion of the resulting damage is expressed
in the title of his book, *Corporate Wives—Corporate Casualties* (Seidenberg,
1973). The spouse and children of workaholics often feel that they come
in second to the job. As one ten-year old daughter explained:

> My Daddy is going to be president of his company one of these
> days. I heard him tell my mother that. He said he had to work day
> and night, but in the end it would be worth it. My mother is not
> so sure . . . and I am not sure, either. My brother and I wish our
> father could be home with us, and not at the office or traveling all
> day and half the night (Machlowitz, 1980, p. 84).

Some superpersons and workaholics are addicted to stress. Job challenges, an over-full schedule, and deadlines serve as stimulants.

Whereas superpersons frequently pay the price through their own burn-out, it is the workaholic's family that succumbs in the workaholism syndrome.

Employer Expectations

Employers frequently expect employees to work more than an eight-hour day or five-day work week. The employee may think that such extra work time and energy are required for career advancement or maybe even to keep the job. The time spent at work reduces time the worker can spend with the family and reduces the amount of time in which to accomplish household tasks or parental or spousal responsibilities. This time squeeze can be a significant source of stress, as family conflict increases and tasks do not get done.

Spouses in either the traditional or the dual-employment pattern may feel that their partner's job requires too much business travel. As family therapists have noted: "A family can be seen as a mobile with the roles and relationships like the strings holding parts together. After regular but long separation, the system is sharply jolted by reentry. But in time, things settle down . . . (with frequent business travel) the family mobile is constantly shaking" (Gullotta & Donohue, 1981, p. 154).

Corporate executive wives have found that they cope better with their husband's travel if they develop interpersonal relationships, establish their own independence and self-sufficiency, and value the corporate lifestyle (Boss, McCubbin, & Lester, 1979). Frequent business travelers have found the following methods to be helpful: warning the family of an impending trip, staying in touch by telephone calls and postcards, tape-recording bedtime stories for the kids before leaving, and taking the family along from time to time (Sullivan, 1980).

Job transfers and relocations are another common employer demand, often included in a promotion. Employers may expect and interpret willingness to relocate as an indication of interest, enthusiasm, and commitment to the company. Families, on the other hand, are likely to be concerned about losing the familiarity of friends, home, stores, and schools, and to question the availability of a job for the spouse and good schools for the children in the new community.

In a recent survey, two-thirds of corporate employers had experienced increased resistance to relocation (Catalyst, 1981). More companies are assisting the spouse of a relocated employee to find a new job. Even so, 15% of relocated spouses must change occupational fields in order to find a job (Brooks, 1981).

The decision not to move may also create work/family stress. Whereas in one family a spouse may blame the partner for problems experienced in moving, in another family the spouse may blame the family's unwillingness to move for holding him/her back and preventing deserved promotions.

Allocation of Time and Energy as a Source of Stress

Like Brett, the corporate manager described at the beginning of this chapter, many people complain that there is never enough time and energy to accomplish all they want to in their work and family roles. As Skinner pointed out in Chapter 6, they experience role overload. This time/energy shortage can be short-term in accomplishing the day-to-day tasks or it can be long-term in accomplishing overall work and family goals. In the short run, couples may develop time management skills and, when financially able, purchase labor-saving devices and hired help. In the longer run, some couples consider role-cycling (Rapoport & Rapoport, 1976), in which each spouse attempts to stagger his or her career progress timetable along with the family's progress. By doing so, they avoid the stress of having demands of both work and family peak during the same period of their lives. For example, when children are very young, one spouse may take a part-time job and then return to full-time work when the children are older and more independent.

At times, however, it is not the amount of time available that creates stress but rather the scheduling of the time. Working an eight-hour evening shift or rotating shift creates different stress than working an eight-hour day shift (Maynard, Maynard, McCubbin, & Shao, 1980). Working evenings or weekends and extensive business travel may make it difficult to spend time with spouse or children when they are not at their own work or school activities (Culbert & Renshaw, 1972).

The time-energy difficulty also partly results from the permeability of boundaries between work and family roles (Pleck, 1977). Thoughts and worries about family intrude into work time and vice versa. The intrusion of family thoughts into work time has been labeled the "fire department ideology of childrearing"—parents at work are in a constant state of preparation for family emergencies such as accidents or illness (Rossi, 1964). On the other hand, even when physically present at home, a family member may be psychologically miles away. Work planning and worries may occupy his or her thoughts even when inappropriate. The inability to concentrate fully on the role one is presently engaged in may create stress for the individual, among family members, or between employer and employee.

Work/family conflicts regarding family roles tend to fall into two areas: allocation of household tasks and child-care responsibilities.

Child-care Responsibilities

Working parents worry about possible negative effects of their working on their children and about choosing and maintaining child-care arrangements.

Many working mothers experience a sense of anxiety or guilt about real or imagined effects of their employment for their children. This feeling is so universal that the magazine *Working Mother* has a monthly column titled "The Guilt Department," which discusses common concerns of working mothers and provides suggestions for coping with time/energy issues.

Research on maternal employment shows, however, that it is how the mother feels about her choice, whether that be going out to work or staying home, that is the strongest influence on the children. In an extensive review of the issue, Hoffman (1974, p. 164) concludes that "the data on the whole suggest that the working mother who obtains personal satisfaction from employment, does not have excessive guilt, and has adequate household arrangements is likely to perform as well as the nonworking mother or better. . . ."

In contrast to the attention paid to maternal employment, the effects of paternal employment on children have been relatively unexplored, most likely due to the implicit assumption that there is no choice—"all men work." It has been suggested that paternity leave, where offered, has been the first policy that legitimizes the shift of some of the father's energies from the workplace to the family (Pleck, 1977). When both maternity and paternity leaves are available to a couple, they are able to share child-care consecutively and the amount of time either parent is gone from the workplace is minimized. Beyond the infant stage of the children's development, an additional advantage for dual-employed couples is that the father and mother tend to discuss and negotiate much more frequently about childrearing issues than traditional couples (Working Family Project, 1978).

Working parents are often told that it is the quality of time, rather than the quantity of time one spends with children, that is significant. Unfortunately, good quality time is difficult to define, to measure, and

to make happen on schedule. Parents who regularly spend uninter-
rupted time with their children, who avoid procrastinating about their
children's needs and wishes, and who provide their children with a
sense of being a high priority are well on their way to having high quality
time (Seiden, 1980). Such parents may find it reassuring to know that,
in a national survey, 87% of teenagers with working parents thought
their mothers spent the right amount of time with them and 64% thought
their fathers did also (General Mills American Family Report, 1981).

Having a good child-care arrangement greatly increases the peace of
mind of a working parent, whether the parent is working out of financial
necessity, to fulfill career goals, to achieve personal satisfaction, or a
combination of these reasons. Considerations of time, cost, reliability,
and distance from home appear to dictate choice of child-care provider
(Rowe, 1978).

Parents have the most difficulty finding and maintaining child-care
when the children are infants, when the children are sick, when school-
age children need care for a short time before and after school, or when
the parents must travel as part of their job. In a recent business-con-
ducted survey, a fourth of the respondents listed child-care problems
as being a detriment to their productivity (Honeywell Women's Task
Force, 1980).

Household Responsibility

A perennial debate for many families concerns who is to do what tasks
in the household. When work demands press into family life, this debate
becomes more complicated. The dispute concerns actual amount of time
spent in housework, as well as attitude regarding who has ultimate
responsibility for the household tasks. Although women have been
changing their traditional roles very rapidly by working outside the
home, men have been slower to change their role within the household.
Time studies indicate that fulltime housewives spend 8.1 hours per day
in household responsibilities, employed wives spend 4.8 hours per day,
but men average only 1.6 hours per day regardless of whether their
wives are employed (Walker & Woods, 1976). This lack of equality can
create problems.

Fueling the debate is the fact that, in many dual-employed families,
the wife retains responsibility for household tasks, even when the husband helps out. She is responsible for orchestrating and monitoring
household functioning. He may feel and is likely to say that he is "helping" her with her responsibility, often to her resentment.

Some couples in these situations reach a compromise by changing expectations: standards about what needs to be done are lowered; husband, children, and hired help do more. Some couples decide that equality of responsibilities on a day-to-day basis is not necessary. Rather, they are concerned with an overall equity, very much dependent on constraints and pressures for each at any particular family stage and career stage (Rapoport & Rapoport, 1975). Flexibility is therefore required as the division of duties are renegotiated as work and family situations change. Many couples find, over time, that they value the increased empathy toward their partner as they both experience household and employment responsibilities.

COPING WITH WORK/FAMILY STRESS

Attitudes and Skills for Families

Several coping strategies effectively employed by families to avoid or relieve work/family stress have been cited in the preceding pages. The idea of *seeking a balance* between work and family demands is central to understanding these coping strategies. The failure to seek a balance is often dysfunctional.

The examples of the workaholic and the superperson were cited earlier. Another example would be the father who fears he will be laid off or fired and then works longer hours to prove his indispensability at work; consequently, he has less time and energy to support his family as they try to deal with the worry about the anticipated loss of his job. Similarly, a worker dissatisfied with his or her job may choose to change careers; but this often results in a drop in income, at least temporarily, or a change in family lifestyle or routine, thereby increasing stress for the family. These situations show how ways of coping with stressors of a feared loss of job or job dissatisfaction can in themselves serve to increase stress in the family system.

But what specific attitudes and skills are useful to families in balancing work life and family life? Agreement between husband and wife on work and family goals is certainly important. Unless husband and wife agree as to the employment pattern they wish to follow and have compatible ideas regarding the most desirable lifestyle, there will be endless conflict. Without such basic compatibility, it is difficult to support the other's goals and activities. Even when both are committed to either a dual-employment or traditional pattern when they marry, there needs to be openness and flexibility as changing needs of the individual or family may dictate a change in employment pattern.

The couple with a mind-set that work/family stressors are challenging rather than simply overwhelming is likely to cope well. They perceive stressful events as "creative disorganization" rather than "disruptive crises" (Hansen & Johnson, 1979) and are better able to tolerate ambiguity. Being able to talk with each other about changing needs, to negotiate, and to compromise is essential. The more open the communication, the more aware the couple becomes of their "tension lines"—the final straw for their tolerance of work/family stressors (Rapoport & Rapoport, 1980).

As Skinner noted in Chapter 6, working families need good time management skills. Saying "no" to low priority requests helps keep obligations and commitments at a manageable level. Allowing less-than-perfect standards for low priority activities increases available time. Being able to compartmentalize work and family roles so that attention is focused on the role presently occupied tends to reduce time required to complete tasks. Being willing and able to delegate some responsibilities and tasks to others, inside or outside the family, lessens pressure.

Turning to others for help is also important. Educational programs and support groups dealing with work/family stressors can help individuals cope with either chronic or acute stressors. By sharing problems in these groups, members often feel relieved when they realize how universal such difficulties are. Group members also share resources for combating the stressor. Such a couples workshop conducted in one corporation had far-reaching consequences: business executives traveled less often, for shorter time periods, and almost never on weekends (Culbert & Renshaw, 1972).

Couples may also find help through books that provide suggestions on how to cope with work/family stressors, ranging from how to evaluate adequate child-care options to how to survive a job transfer.

Employing organizations can also be helpful if the employees ask for assistance. The employee request is necessary, however, since, for example, 29% of companies in one survey said they would be likely to assist in finding employment for the spouse of a relocating employee if the employee requested it (Catalyst, 1981).

Workplace Policies for Family Coping

Thus far, this chapter has focused on work/family stressors as they affect the family. These same work/family stressors affect an employee's performance at work, as the case example at the start of the chapter showed. Meisha's family responsibilities were interfering with her work and jeopardizing her job.

Employers are increasingly considering policies and programs to reduce work/family stress. A recent survey of corporations indicated that concern for problems of two-earner families was motivated by an awareness that such problems affected recruiting, employee morale, productivity, and ultimately corporate profits (Catalyst, 1981). Child-care problems contribute to increased tardiness, absenteeism, turnover and restrictions on business traveling (Honeywell Women's Task Force, 1980).

Corporate response tends to occur in three phases. Initially, concern is with identifying work/family stressors and making policy and program recommendations. Then personnel managers, often in conjunction with interested employees, determine how to implement recommended policies and programs, such as work scheduling flexibility, child-care options, educational assistance and fringe benefit programs. Finally, an assessment is made to see whether the intended results of the policy actually materialized and if there were any unintended consequences. A job applicant interested in reducing work/family stress would do well to check benefits and policies of a prospective employer.

Flexibility in work scheduling is, for many, a highly valued work policy. In the most widely publicized variation, flextime, the worker can begin and end the day at a time convenient for himself or herself. The flextime schedule has two basic elements. First, there is a common core time, say from 10 a.m. to 3 p.m., when all workers are required to be on the job. Second, there is a flexible period of time at each end of the workday during which workers can choose their own arrival and departure times. This flexibility in workday scheduling enables the worker to establish a work schedule allowing more freedom of options for family and personal time. Required or desired activities, such as dentist's appointments or children's school plays, can be attended to during normal work hours. Some families where both parents have flextime arrange their work schedules so one parent is at home in the morning before the children leave for school and one parent is home in the afternoon when they return from school.

Flexibility of work site provides similar advantages. When employees can do part or all of their work at home, they have more opportunity to coordinate the timing of work and family activities in a desirable fashion. Other rearranged work week alternatives with possible advantages for families include compressing the work week into four 10-hour days, two people sharing one job, and permanent part-time employment.

The work/family stresses and needs of families with children are increasingly being addressed by corporate programs and policies. Maternity leave policies are commonplace and more companies are considering paternity leave policies. Many companies are recognizing and not penalizing their employees for the fact that sick days are being used for their children's illnesses as well as their own.

Recognizing that difficulties in child-care arrangements provide distractions for many of their employees, companies have attempted a variety of solutions: establishment of on-site child-care facilities; reserving slots in existing child-care facilities close to the work site in order to ensure availability of child-care to employees; developing a community-wide child-care information and referral service; offering child-care vouchers as an employee benefit. Suitability of any particular child-care solution depends on factors such as size of the company, percentage of parents in their work force, degree of centralization of the work force, and extent of existing child-care facilities in the community.

Some companies are providing seminars about parent-child relationships and parenting to their employees. The Texas Family Institute, for example, regularly contracts with companies for a series of noon-hour sessions held at the work site. In considering what the content of such a series should be, a report by Honeywell, Inc. suggested these topics: finding, selecting and evaluating child-care; identifying resources which can assist working parents; building children's self-esteem, independence, and ability to assume responsibility; making the most of time available to spend with family members; understanding and coping with work/family conflicts; effective time management at work and at home (Honeywell Working Parents' Task Force, 1981).

Some companies serve an information and referral function, letting employees know of resources available through community groups, educational institutions, or social service agencies. This safeguards them from being accused of paternalism if they provide an extensive employee assistance program or of being discriminatory if funds are expended for services for working parent employees that are not appropriate for non-parents.

With the increasing number of two-earner couples, more families are finding that fringe benefits such as family medical insurance are duplicated by their two employers. Some companies have begun to offer a "cafeteria style" benefits program in which employees may select from a range of benefits those most valuable to them. For example, in lieu of medical insurance already provided by the spouse's employers, one person may decide to take a child-care voucher. Another may opt for an education voucher, when the employer pays the cost of degree-related coursework.

Fringe benefit programs of other companies take into account the special characteristics of their work force. For example, an organization which has had a stable work force for many years may have many employees approaching retirement age who would find it helpful if the company were to offer flexible or part-time employment opportunities for older workers so that they can ease into retirement. Pre-retirement seminars may also be offered which focus on psychological, financial, and health issues of retirement. An organization with a young work force is more likely to be concerned with child-care options. An organization having many employees from two-earner families might want to develop a consistent relocation service available to people being transferred.

What becomes evident from these many possible employer responses to work/family stress is that there is no one overall solution. As one employee said, "You know, help with any one of the problems of working parents (employees) is help with all of them. They all overlap and they all influence each other" (Oser, 1980, p. 4).

Although a great number of work/family stressors have been identified in this chapter, the purpose has not been to paint a picture of gloom and doom. The more roles one occupies, the more likely it is that one will experience friction from conflicting demands. But because work and family roles are both so crucial for many people, there is a continuing search for and discovery of new coping strategies. The challenge becomes developing one's lifestyle and selecting one's coping mechanisms so that the balance between work life and family life is satisfying.

12

Societal Stress: The Black Family

HARRIETTE P. McADOO

A group of Black parents were discussing their children's experiences of racism. One father said, "When Marcia was three, we were at a shopping plaza and an older white child taunted her about being Black. Marcia didn't know what to say, and walked off. When we talked to her about it, she seemed to feel better, and I had hoped she would forget all about it. But she didn't—it still bothers her, she still remembers it." Another parent said, "I know my kids aren't treated the same as whites at school. Somehow, you know, teachers seem to expect less from Black kids. The kids feel it, and wonder why they're treated differently."

These parents are painfully aware of the stress of racism in their lives and their children's lives. Being a member of a minority group in America means being treated differently, and this societal stressor places huge demands on family life.

Until recently, both family scholars and the public have attributed racial differences in family life to the poverty in which many Black families live. Once Blacks were better educated and upwardly mobile, so the theory went, these differences would disappear. But the civil rights movement and the development of group consciousness among people of color brought to reality the fact that Blacks were not being allowed to melt into a single white American culture. They were actively affirming their pride in their unique African-American heritage and demanding an end to racial discrimination. Although some assimilation has occurred, differences persist in religion, music, and language, pointing to the basic soul-searching role that cultural heritage plays in the maintenance of positive self-identity and positive mental health. These cultural differences tend to persist even when Black families become part of the middle class (McAdoo, 1979).

Of course, Black families share many characteristics and problems with white families: The developmental changes in children and parents as they grow and age; the problems of single parents or dual-employed families; the stressors of inflation, unemployment, war or natural disasters—all of these are discussed in detail in other chapters of these volumes and all have relevance for Black families. But they must be seen in context: A racist environment changes and intensifies the meaning and impact of these normative and catastrophic sources of stress. Black families are not able to have the same opportunities and experiences as white families, and these differences are important reasons for considering their special stressors and coping patterns.

The focus of this chapter is on the societal stressors of racism on Black families, and how these families remain strong and responsive as they cope with these stressors. This chapter will sketch some of the stressors of racism by discussing the concept of mundane extreme environmental stress and by looking specifically at how this environment affects the economic situation of Black families. The second part of the chapter deals with how the special strengths of Black families contribute to their ability to cope with these stressors; the reliance on the extended family and community for support and the flexibility of roles in the family are two such strengths.

STRESSORS OF RACISM: THE MUNDANE
EXTREME ENVIRONMENT

Chester Pierce, a Black psychiatrist, has compared the stress on Blacks in the United States with the harsh physical stress on those who live in extreme climates. Just as the day-to-day demands of coping with severe cold and scarce food supply define life for the Eskimo people in the Arctic, so severe racial prejudice defines life for Blacks. Pierce (1975), borrowing a term from anthropologists, calls this racist "climate" a *mundane extreme environment*. In this case the extreme environment is not a physical, geographic one, but a social one; it provides the entire context for people's lives and expectations (Peters, 1981). The "extreme" difficulties which white society imposes on Black people by denying their identity, their values, and their economic opportunity are not unusual or extraordinary but "mundane," daily pressures for Blacks.

The concept of a mundane extreme environment suggests vividly how racism is a pervasive, daily reality for Black families. This reality goes beyond the single interactions with non-Blacks in the neighborhood or with strangers on the way to school or work, when a Black child or adult may be treated differently than one who is non-Black. It even goes beyond the cross burnings that are increasing and the actual violence that occurs more frequently than we would like to admit. Rather, the reality for Black individuals is affected most seriously by the negative perceptions that are held about them by whites. These negative images are part of the American culture and difficult to escape, for they are projected continuously throughout the culture—through TV, through pictures in school books, in ethnic jokes, and from personal experiences when the different racial groups come into contact with each other. These attitudes come to the surface when there is a lack of acceptance for those with cultural differences, or when teachers do not expect as much from their Black children and, therefore, are given less in return. It occurs also when employers do not consider Blacks to be capable of doing a job regardless of their individual abilities or training.

It is important to see that the subordinate social position of Black Americans is supported and maintained by social institutions such as schools or the social welfare system (Ogbu, 1978). We must avoid "blaming the victims" of this pervasive, extremely stressful environment. While degrees of racial oppression vary with each situation, the potential for being devalued and put down is *always* present, dangling constantly over Blacks, beyond their control.

Economic Stressors

One of the most basic ways this stressful environment affects families is in the denial of economic opportunities. This denial manifests itself in the inadequate education, job discrimination, and higher unemployment rates, all resulting in lower incomes for Black families.

Unemployment

The editors of these volumes have chosen to classify the stressors of unemployment as a "catastrophe"; however, unemployment for Black urban youth is such a common experience that it is often seen in the Black community as a "normative" stressor. While the white unemployed youth can be confident that the catastrophe of unemployment is for a limited time, the Black youth in the same situation knows that he probably will face it for an extended time. Due to the problems of poor education and limited employment opportunities, families of color in all social classes have, in general, lower incomes than white families, even when they have college degrees. Forty-one percent of Black children live in families with poverty level incomes, many headed by single mothers (Pearce & McAdoo, 1981). Some say that all of these conditions are the result of things that are wrong with Blacks themselves. A more accurate analysis reveals these stressful conditions to be the result of a long continuing history of inequities that have fostered the development of groups who do not develop the skills or who lack the social and personal connections that would allow them to be able to help themselves out of their impoverished situations.

One cannot help but respond in amazement that there still exists the energy among Blacks to attempt to be self-sufficient, when there have been so many barriers placed before them. For example, one of the strongest values that Black families have had is faith that education would improve their situation (McAdoo, 1978). During the first years of elementary school, the parents have high expectations of their children and high dreams for them. While the parents are dreaming of their children bettering their lives and having less stress than they themselves have had, others are viewing these high expectations as "unrealistic." What happens is that teachers really do not expect their students in urban schools to achieve and send them the unspoken messages that they really are not expected to achieve. As a result, the students live up to the lowered expectations and another class of students becomes unable to compete in the labor market.

Although minority enrollment in colleges and universities has risen dramatically in the last 10 years, most minority students in school beyond high school have been enrolled in terminal or community college programs. Blacks have traditionally been denied access to higher education related to technology, business, and sciences in four-year universities, and thus, to the higher-paying jobs that follow. Even now, most minority students are concentrated in a few two-year colleges, while whites go to universities (Institute for the Study of Educational Policy, 1980). Black students withdraw from these institutions at a much higher rate than do whites. Few Blacks go into the engineering or other technical fields which command the highest salaries on graduation (McAdoo, 1982a).

But even with a degree, racial discrimination on the job is a reality. Minority college graduates can expect to earn only 85% of what white men with similar backgrounds earn. A 1980 *Wall Street Journal* article reports that Black middle managers feel that racism continues to bar them from promotions and the accompanying higher salaries (Kaufman, 1980). In one study of middle-class Black families, many parents reported experiencing insidious or overt discrimination at work which hindered job advancement (McAdoo, 1979).

The national unemployment rate for Blacks is twice the rate for whites (McAdoo, 1982a). For young Black men in urban areas, the situation is desperate; recent data indicate the national youth unemployment rate among Blacks is nearly 60%. Even this number, appalling as it is, is probably too low, for it only counts those who consistently look for jobs; millions of young people have simply given up. According to Jones (1971), these teenagers have become permanent members of the underclass, whose prospects are worse now than they were for anyone during the Great Depression of the 1930s. These young men will enter middle adulthood with no work experience; this extended unemployment will permanently affect their earning potential.

White youth who are unemployed for periods of time probably live at home where at least one parent has a job. Black youth, in contrast, often live in a one-parent household with a mother who is under economic stress. U. S. Census and Department of Labor data show that 40% of these unemployed youth have no relative who is working. Not only do they not have a job, but many are also without a realistic role model of an actively employed adult.

Another factor in explaining the generally lower income levels of Black families is the higher proportion of single-parents and thus single wage-earner families. Half of all Black families are single-parent families headed by women, partly because there are fewer men than women, and partly because of the increase in divorces and teen pregnancies. Many of these women-headed Black families have incomes below the poverty line; Black single mothers are less likely than whites to be collecting child support or alimony, and far fewer have jobs (McAdoo, 1982a). Yet the majority of Black parents are self-supporting and not dependent on public support.

Housing

The lower economic status of Blacks has potentially stressful ripple effects for families. The cost of housing, for example, may restrict them to living in high-crime neighborhoods or public housing projects. For example, Ruby Jones and her three children live in a two-story cement block apartment building in a housing project built in the 1950s. It was built in an industrial area near the center of the city. Two years ago, some of the units were torn down when the state widened the freeway, and the roar of the traffic goes on all the time. "It's a messed-up place to live," says Ruby. "There is a shooting or fire here almost every week, sometimes two or three a week. My kids can hear the shots and sirens when they are doing their homework or trying to sleep at night. I'm embarrassed to say we live here." Although Ruby likes her neighbors and has a brother living nearby, she wishes she could earn enough money to afford a better home for her kids, but rents are too high everywhere else.

Health Care

Reduced income for minority families also affects the quality of health care for Black families. Poor families avoid the expenses of preventative health care, and as inflation hits middle-income families harder, they begin to shift priorities too (General Mills American Family Report, 1979). Concentrated in low-level jobs with poor benefits, Black families are less likely than whites to have adequate health insurance; surveys of Black families indicate that they tend to feel that their health care is poor (McAdoo, 1982b). The infant mortality rate for Blacks is 21.7 per 1000 births, as compared to 12.3 for whites. This higher rate probably indicates poor health care during pregnancy, resulting in low birth weights and more birth defects. The proportion of Black children who have not been immunized against infectious diseases has risen recently, leading to fears of renewed outbreaks of these diseases. The overall mortality rate for Blacks has been consistently higher than for whites, and a recent survey of Black parents found that many partially attributed this higher death rate to the psychological and social pressures of racism in their everyday environment (McAdoo, 1982b).

These stressors, both overt and covert, form the most difficult barrier preventing Blacks from living without a high degree of stress. The stressors of discrimination and of lower economic status result in living conditions that are unhealthy, but these environments are blamed upon the persons who are really the victims, rather than the sources of these stresses. The mundane stressful environments are the result of discrimination that interacts with people who have been made to feel that there is only limited hope for bettering their lives, and thus this environment is perpetuated.

COPING WITH THE STRESSORS OF RACISM

These stressors of racism and economic disadvantage do indeed create an extreme environment for Black families. Yet it would be wrong to view these families as totally unhealthy or inadequate because of these stressors. In fact, the family has remained a strong and responsible institution for Black people throughout their history, even during the slavery era (Staples, 1971).

The most functional and effective coping strategies for Blacks come from the strength and support they find within their own families and kin networks. The strengths we will discuss here are the reliance on the help-exchange network of family and friends, and the flexibility of family roles in Black families.

The Help-exchange Network of Family and Friends

William, age 32, and Gloria Robinson, age 28, live in a large midwestern city near her parents and four of her six brothers and sisters. They have two small children. William is a carpenter, although he has been laid off for the past two months. His unemployment checks sometimes do not quite cover expenses, and he is sometimes depressed that he can't find another job. When their car broke down last month, they borrowed the money for the repair bill from William's brother. Gloria herself has been able to pick up some temporary work, mostly through an employment agency. While she is working and William is not, the kids stay with Gloria's sister Donna. The two sisters often help each other with child-care responsibilities. Last year Gloria's sister Jane and Jane's daughter lived with William and Gloria for several months while Jane looked for a new job and apartment. Gloria sees her sisters often, sometimes two or three times a week, and the whole family gets together at her parents' house almost every weekend. When she is worried about money or has an argument with William, she turns to her sisters and her mother.

In Gloria's case, her family is her main source of social support, with some help from William's family. They help when her nuclear family needs money, when she needs a babysitter, or when she just wants someone to talk to. The family members see one another frequently, and Gloria gives help as well as receiving it. Sociologists term this arrangement a "kin help-exchange network." In Gloria's case "kin" refers to her parents and siblings. For other Black families the term can include more distant relatives, as well as family friends or neighbors (Stack, 1975; Staples, 1971). Census data indicate that Black families take in relatives to live in their households for a time much more often than white families (Billingsley, 1968; Hill, 1971). Black parents report feeling more protective of their children than white parents do. They often act as a buffer between their children and the racism of teachers or other whites. Black childrearing patterns reflect this "buffering"; parents actively promote their children's psychological well-being in the face of omnipresent stressors (Nobles, 1974; Richardson, 1981). To cope with a hostile society, Black families have turned to the resources within their families and among their friends.

Nor is this reliance on support from kin merely a response to poverty. A study of stress and coping patterns of middle-class Black families found that almost every family gave and received help from their kin network (McAdoo, 1982b). This help took the form of child-care, loans of money in emergencies, emotional support, and exchange of help with repairs or chores. Those who were under more stress relied on kin the most.

These middle-class parents were aware of the sacrifices their families had made to put them through school and help them succeed, and they regarded their own success as an achievement shared with the wider kin group. They felt, in turn, that offering help and support was "what is done in families" and valued their extended family relations very highly. Although few actually shared housing with extended family members, most lived close by. This study revealed that these families showed a strong preference for handling stress within the family and would turn to an outside agency only when they had exhausted their internal resources (McAdoo, 1979).

The strong commitment to the success of their children and the pride in educational accomplishments which the subjects of McAdoo's study felt in their families and which other studies have found (Peters, 1976) may reflect a coping strategy. Hope for the future of the children may help parents to maintain optimism in the face of current difficulties or hardships. As one parent said, "My parents struggled to put us through school; it seemed to make up for the choices they never had" (McAdoo, 1979).

Black families also get support from the broader Black community. Although religion is less important than it used to be for many families, churches do provide spiritual, psychological, and material help. Pride in the Black heritage is another functional coping strategy, in that it strengthens self-esteem; families develop a positive sense of the value of their diverse African-American experiences and try to pass this on to their children (McAdoo, 1978; Staples, 1971). The study of middle-class family stress and coping found that parents under greater stress were more likely to be involved in integrated or all-white social groups; lower-stressed parents were more active in all-Black social activities (McAdoo, 1982b). Parents who cope most successfully seem to maintain a balance between their economic aspirations, found in the white world, and their roots in the Black community. This necessary *duality* of Black life is experienced by many as another source of stress.

Flexibility of Family Roles

In white families, the roles of each parent and of the children are clearly and, until recently, rigidly defined: father was the breadwinner, while mother tended to care for the home and children. But in Black families, both parents have always had to work outside of the home just to make ends meet; the dual-employed couple is not a new phenomenon among Blacks. Both parents share the task of earning a living and share the domestic and childrearing tasks as well.

For example, George Bradley is an assistant city clerk. His wife Mary works the second shift at a large computer manufacturing company. While she sees the children off to school, she still has time to take care of the shopping and do some housecleaning before she leaves for work. George gets dinner for the kids, helps them with their homework, and enjoys watching TV with them before he puts them to bed. Larry, their 16-year-old, is in charge if George must work late, and the other two have their assigned chores around the house.

This pattern is becoming familiar in many white families too. But George and Mary grew up in households like this and are comfortable with these flexible roles. Research into Black families shows that most marriages are egalitarian; that is, husband and wife share authority to make decisions and share family responsbilities (Hill, 1971; Hyman & Reed, 1969; Mack, 1971). Black men are not threatened by the fact that their wives work outside of the home as some white men are; that is the pattern they expect and are accustomed to (Peters, 1976; Tenhouten, 1970). This role flexibility and shared decision-making ease strains in dual-employed and dual-career families. Moreover, Black women are less "helpless" if they are divorced or widowed and are better able to deal with the role changes required in the transition to a single-parent family or stepfamily. This flexibility of roles, too, serves to complement the support of the extended family; for example, it allows for entrance of other relatives into the nuclear family unit.

CONCLUSION

In this chapter, the stressors of the "mundane extreme environment" generated by racism are discussed briefly, with an emphasis on those associated with the economic disadvantages many Blacks face. But the strengths and coping strategies of Black families have helped them to handle this "extreme environment." Reliance on family and friends—the help-exchange kin network—and the capacity for flexibility in family roles are two such strengths that have been among the most effective coping strategies.

These aspects of Black family stress and coping have important implications for public policy, as well as for family stress theory and research. Social service agencies should try to increase and support the existing helping networks rather than replace them. One example of how this has been encouraged were the tax reforms that permitted deductions for child-care payments to grandparents. At the same time, policymakers should not assume the Black families will "take care of their own" so well that they do not need services. They should, rather, be aware of the great diversity of experiences and needs in Black families and avoid stereotyping—even stereotyping that is positive (McAdoo, 1979).

Obviously, a serious commitment to work with Black families, or with minority families in general, calls for interventions at what Melson (Chapter 10) calls the exosystem (the Black community and the larger social context), as well as the microsystem (the Black family unit and kin). The roots of social discrimination and mundane stressors must be attacked and eliminated and, therefore, need to be targets of social policy and concern, even though the fruits of our interventions will not be seen for at least another decade. Concomitantly, we need to advance our understanding of family coping within the family-kin network, with the expectation that such knowledge can be used to strengthen Black families now and in the future.

CHAPTER

13

Environmental Stress: The Rural Family

RAYMOND T. COWARD and
ROBERT W. JACKSON

> Jim, 14, drove the tractor towards the fields on the farm his family
> owned with his uncle. An early June hailstorm had flattened most of
> their 1,600 acres of young corn; while the family had government
> insurance to cover the financial loss, he couldn't help feeling angry
> and frustrated at their bad luck. He had overheard his parents talking
> about selling their share of the farm: High interest rates on money
> needed to buy equipment, seed, and fertilizer, low crop prices,
> restrictions on grain sales due to international politics, and now bad
> weather made it tough to keep ahead as a farmer. Three years ago,
> his mother had taken a job in the nearest big town to bring in some
> extra income. It seemed his family had to deal with one problem after
> another.

One does not automatically associate this kind of stress with rural life.
Popular images depict family life in small towns and rural America as
slow-paced, peaceful, tranquil, and undisturbed—a throwback to earlier,
less complicated times free of the hustle, bustle, and pollution of the

cities. Impressions seem caught in the sepia tones of early photographs or cast in the monolithic caricatures that novelists created of the first settlers of the plains. Rural America is still often lauded as the "backbone of this country," embodying the most honorable values of man—honesty, hard work, self-reliance, and independence. It is seen as a healthy environment in which to raise children and a place where the ties of family and friendship are valued, maintained, and enriched. Most Americans report that they would prefer to live in nonmetropolitan communities or areas that are a distance from central cities (Blackwood & Carpenter, 1978).

In reality, however, family life in rural America is seldom so pristine. For millions of rural residents, life is shaped and molded by harsh circumstances that sometimes severely threaten the fabric of their existence. Less well understood and acknowledged in popular accounts of rural life are the following observations:

- Rural residents experience a greater incidence, prevalence and severity of malnutrition than their urban counterparts;
- almost one-half of all occupied substandard housing and about two-thirds of all houses without adequate plumbing are located in rural communities;
- rural families have the nation's highest rates of maternal and infant mortality;
- unemployment and underemployment rates are higher for rural than for urban areas;
- the rate of increase in divorces in rural areas exceeds that of metropolitan America;
- whereas one in nine urban residents lives below the poverty line, one in six rural residents is in the same situation; and
- government studies reveal that many rural underground water sources are contaminated and rural drinking water is less likely to meet federal bacteriological requirements.

Nevertheless, this sobering list does not mean that life in small towns has disintegrated totally or that we have been the targets of some deliberate propaganda campaign. These facts should, however, reshape our idyllic notions so they resemble reality more closely. Many of the social forces that have molded and recast the lives of urban families in the past quarter of a century are paralleled in rural and small town families. At the same time, family life in rural society continues to be significantly different from urban life in many socioeconomic characteristics and interpersonal processes (Coward & Smith, 1981). Coward (1981, p. 18) has suggested that it is as if "rural and urban families are riding parallel but different roads . . . heading in the same direction but remaining on separate paths." Carlson, Lassey, and Lassey (1981, p. 60) characterized the difference as ". . . more a matter of rapidity and degree than of change versus nonchange."

In the sections that follow we will illustrate some of the rapidly changing dimensions of family life in rural America, particularly focusing on three sets of external factors associated with greater stress: (a) economic and employment stressors; (b) community stressors; and (c) environmental stressors. In later sections of the chapter we will examine the context in which rural families attempt to cope with these stressors and the policy implications of these conditions. First, let us turn our attention to the continued importance of the rural sector to our country.

RURAL AMERICA: WHERE IS IT? WHY IS IT IMPORTANT?

More than 50 definitions of rurality are currently established by federal governmental and legislative regulations and at least that many can be identified in the professional research literature. Nevertheless, to paraphrase Atchley (1975), no one disputes that there are rural areas of our country and that families live there; what is debated is the precise boundaries of those categories, not their existence. Residence is not a dichotomy, but a *continuum* that contains on one end New York City, San Francisco, and Atlanta and at the other extreme such places as Beanblossom, Indiana, Deer Lodge, Montana, and Walnut Ridge, Arkansas.

The decade of the 1970s has been called a "renaissance" for rural America because the well-established pattern of rural to urban migration was reversed. Data from the 1980 Census indicate that, in all regions of the nation except the South, the rate of growth in nonmetropolitan communities exceeded that of metropolitan areas in the preceding decade (Beale, 1981). This trend is interesting to family sociologists because it reflects a search for a better quality of life rather than perceived opportunities for prosperity or escape from economic hardship, political persecution, or famine.

Although this migrational reversal is important in both symbolic and real terms, it should not overshadow the already significantly large, stable rural population that exists. Nationally the vast majority of people who lived in small towns and rural communities at the time of the 1980

Census had lived in similar areas a decade before. By 1980 the total rural population had topped 62 million—one out of every four Americans (U.S. Department of Agriculture, 1981).*

These migrational forces have joined with other economic, political and sociocultural factors to transform rural America. Change is a central theme for all rural Americans—change in themselves, in their families, and in the communities in which they live. Coward (1981, p. 20) has suggested that "a changing rural society is affecting the family . . . and the changing family is affecting rural society." The resulting synergism is, for many rural families, potentially stressful.

STRESSORS IN THE RURAL ENVIRONMENT

Many of the stressors discussed throughout this book are not bound by geographic area or associated with particular residential districts. No family is immune to the stress associated with normative transitions that characterize the life cycle—coupling or parenthood, for example (see Chapters 2, 4, 5). Likewise, some of the catastrophic life stressors —prolonged illness, rape, or sudden divorce—are not confined to families in urban or rural settings (see Volume II). Some stressors, however, e.g., poverty, are more prevalent in rural areas, while other stressors, e.g., crime, are less prevalent. Still others, such as social isolation, are made more severe due to the unique circumstances and physical environment of rural life. Indeed, the ecological approach to the study of behavior emphasizes the close association between people and their environment and the influence of the physical environment on human interaction. Ford (1978, p. 4) noted that ". . . human ecologists see social forms arising from and modified by human cultural adaptation to environmental circumstances." For him and other proponents of human ecology, the continued appreciable differences between the city and the country (with respect to geography, population density, building construction, and other significant factors that comprise the environment) result in continued differences in social life and family interaction. The legitimacy of this theoretical approach has been advanced recently by

---

*The traditional U.S. Census definition of rural includes those residents of open country and towns of less than 2,500 population. The metropolitan-nonmetropolitan distinction has also been frequently used in literature. Nonmetropolitan residents are individuals who live outside a county or group of contiguous counties in which there is at least one city, or twin cities, with a population of 50,000 or more.

the efforts of scientists in the areas of social ecology and environmental psychology.

In the sections below we discuss three categories of stressors outside the family that are significant in shaping the character of family life in contemporary rural America. Each of these illustrates the interplay between environment and behavior.

Economic and Employment Stressors

Family stress caused by insufficient financial resources is well documented and accepted (see Chapter 12). Prolonged economic hardship causes personal disruption and interpersonal strife and extracts a substantial toll. What is less understood, among the general public as well as among academicians, is the large proportion of the rural population which exists in poverty. Poverty is often considered an urban problem which haunts the back alleys and housing projects of our inner cities. It is true that in absolute numbers there are more poor families in America's cities; yet, a significant percentage of the nation's poor—40% in 1978—live in rural areas. Furthermore, a proportionally greater percentage of the *rural* population lives in poverty—13.5% in 1978, in contrast to 10.4% of the urban population (National Rural Center, 1981).

As policymakers and service providers attempt to respond to the needs of the poor, they must not forget the prevalence and effect of this malady on small towns and rural communities. In a background paper developed by the National Rural Center (1981), policymakers were reminded of the following circumstances:*

- Of the over nine million rural poor, approximately seven million were white and more than two million were Black (including a total of 508,000 Hispanics in both groups). Rural Black families were three times as likely to be poor as rural white families.
- 27% of rural white families and 56% of rural Black families had incomes of less than $10,000 a year—below or just barely above the poverty level.
- The majority of the rural poor lived in husband-wife households—61% as opposed to 38% in urban areas. This is an important consideration in those states that limit public assistance programs to single-parent households.

---

*Unless otherwise noted, all the statistics for this section are for the year 1978.

- Approximately one of every five rural poor families relied totally on their earnings to meet their needs and received no public assistance or other transfer of income. Conversely, approximately one-third of the rural poor relied totally on income other than earnings, including Social Security, public assistance and supplemental security income. The remaining families had an income that was a mixture of earnings and transfer income.

In addition to those living below poverty guidelines, larger segments of the populations of small towns and rural communities (as compared to urban cities) are unemployed, underemployed, and seasonally employed. Each of these patterns can produce an unstable, fluctuating, and stressful family environment. Although many of these families are able to "make do" because of their own individual tenacity and ingenuity, the eventual toll on the family unit should not be ignored or underestimated.

These patterns of economic uncertainty have been persistent in some chronically depressed rural areas (e.g., Appalachia and the Southern Delta) and, therefore, have affected several generations of the same family. Some sociologists believe that the value and belief systems that emerge under such prolonged hardships can eventually serve to perpetuate poverty by providing a false sense of well-being and security for the family while encouraging acceptance and compliance (Fitchen, 1981).

The recent past has seen an enormous shift in the employment patterns of rural Americans. It is no longer accurate to use "rural" to mean "agriculture." According to U.S. Bureau of the Census (1978) figures, by 1977 there were almost three times as many factory workers as farm workers in rural America, and only 8.6% of the rural population was employed in farming categories (including forestry and fisheries). This shift has caused a whole generation of rural Americans to be transformed from an agriculturally dominated culture to a more diverse economic complex.

The simultaneous decline in the number of family owned and operated farms has been astonishing. Wilkening (1981, p. 28) noted that from "a peak of 6.8 million farms in 1935, the number has declined to 2.7 million in 1977." While the number of family farms has declined, the average size of individual operations has increased about 150% and the capital investment necessary to operate these larger units has risen markedly. Many of those farmers with small operations who have managed to remain in agriculture have been forced to find work off the farm.

Wilkening (1981) stated that by 1978 over half of the male farm operators in America were also employed off the farm. At this time, we can only speculate about how stressful it is for the family that can't make a living doing what it wants to do—farm the land—but must find off-farm employment because the farm operation doesn't generate enough income or requires a prohibitive overhead investment.

Finally, for families, perhaps the most significant change in the rural economy has been the number of women taking out-of-the-home jobs. During the decade of the 1970s the paid labor force participation of rural women increased by 53%—4.5 million more rural women accepted employment outside the home (Bescher-Donnelly & Smith, 1981). These same authors estimated that by 1980 almost 48% of all nonmetropolitan women were employed. The potential for stress in dual-employment families is discussed elsewhere (see Chapter 6), but is perhaps made worse in rural families because there are fewer child-care facilities in small towns and because dual employment deviates from the traditional rural family norms and expectations (Coward, 1982).

Community Stressors

There is a great diversity among the many geographically separate rural areas of our country. Though small towns have much in common, they are not carbon copies of one another. The two community stressors discussed below—dependency ratios and sudden economic development—are relevant to many, but not all, rural towns.

Dependency Ratio. The *dependency ratio* is a measure of the percentage of people in a community who are either over 65 or under 18 years of age, as compared to the number of individuals in all other age categories. It is referred to as the "dependency" ratio because these two periods of the life span are times when dependence on others is generally the greatest. Rural areas tend to have higher dependency ratios. That is, compared to cities and suburbs, a significantly larger percentage of the rural population is made up of people under 18 and over 65. Each of these age periods traditionally have been linked to higher levels of family stress.

Moreover, a higher dependency ratio holds the potential for generating community level stress. Dependent individuals in these age categories contribute *less* to the economy of the local community than people in the prime of their earning power, yet they require *more* community services (e.g., education, health and human services) than do their fellow residents. This can cause a tax burden on local rural communities as they attempt to generate the revenue for needed services. Conversely, an inadequate revenue base can result in a narrower range and lower quality of services or even the total absence of some necessary services. Each of these scenarios may increase stress for individual families.

Sudden Economic Development. Some rural communities have been caught in the whirlwind development of the "energy vortex." Small villages and remote wilderness areas of Alaska and the continental Far West have been swept into the mad-dash search for new energy sources. Sometimes this development is well planned and thought out and both preserves the integrity of the native environment and protects the interests of the local residents. More often the process resembles the frontier "boom town." The resulting cultural clash and rapidity of change bring about increased stress for both the indigenous residents and the newcomers (Uhlmann, 1981). Community leaders and individual families are sometimes caught between the conflicting goals of maximal growth and minimal structural and environmental damage, while building a base for long-term economic stability. Families become stressed as they try to keep the lifestyles they value while taking advantage of the newly created opportunities.

When economic growth and development come to rural regions, prosperity has not always been equally distributed among all segments of the society. Reflecting on the industrial revitalization that the South enjoyed in the 1970s, one Black community action worker reminded a group of academics that there were some shady spots in the Sun Belt. He argued that the poorest families and the most economically depressed rural communities were often the last to share in the newfound wealth of a region (Farmer, 1981).

Environmental Stressors

The complex interaction between population sparsity, distance, and topography can create a considerable degree of isolation for rural residents. This aloneness and tranquility are the legend of rural life and contribute heavily to subjective measures of the quality of life, but this same isolation is the essence of "cabin fever" and can bring on severe periods of depression and create frighteningly lonely social islands during periods of personal or family stress.

Isolation can be complicated by extreme weather conditions and geographic location. For example, by Western Montana standards, most of the travel distances in the Northeast are within reason if not miniscule. Yet, a distance of seven or eight miles on a back, mountain pass road, in the middle of a Vermont winter or during mud season, might as well be ten times that distance.

Indeed, the lives of rural Americans are intimately entwined with, and thus vulnerable to, the weather. A higher proportion of rural workers are involved in industries affected by weather—agriculture, fishing, mining, forestry, wildlife management, and recreation. Every year there are some farmers who are devastated by droughts, floods, tornadoes, or hailstorms. The low snowfall of the winter of 1980 meant severe economic hardship for the thousands of rural residents who work in towns and industries in ski areas. Hardship is also, in part, a function of the interaction between weather, topography, and distance. Rural schools close more often because of weather, rural roads are impassable during certain parts of the year, electrical outages are more common, and rural family life seems to follow the ebb and tide of weather fluctuations.

THE CONTEXT OF COPING

Another popular image of the rural family portrait is the family immersed in a strong and pervasive social support network of kin, friends, and church. Maguire (1980, p. 42) described these naturally occurring systems as "preventive forces or buffers" that help people cope with "transition, stress, physical problems and social emotional problems without resorting to the still somewhat stigmatized formal social services." It is the general impression that rural communities rally around individuals and families during times of crisis and are prepared to respond to their various needs.

Unfortunately, there is little empirical support for this folklore. To the extent that kin, friends, and neighbors can serve to support families during periods of stress, the conclusion to be drawn from the research literature is that rural families are not particularly more advantaged. Lee and Cassidy (1981, p. 51) concluded that:

> . . . there is not much difference in frequency of interaction with kin between rural and urban residents. Theories which imply that such differences do exist, at least in the contemporary United States, need careful scrutiny and qualification in light of the empirical evidence.

Factors other than residence seem to be more powerful in predicting whether a family will have a strong support network of family and community. The apparent "friendliness" of many small towns is not necessarily the same as "support" in times of family crisis.

If rural families do not have significantly different informal supports available to them, what about the formal support systems that are available? In this area the data are clear—rural health and human services are less abundant, less accessible, and more expensive per unit to deliver than in urban areas. This pattern is persistent across a range of services and includes professional helpers such as physicians, social workers, child-care providers, service providers for the aged, and mental health workers. These discrepancies in services have diminished somewhat in recent years, but the development and delivery of sufficient services for the rural family in crisis remain a crucial challenge.

We can now conclude that the rural family is not necessarily advantaged with the availability of informal social support and is distinctly disadvantaged with respect to access to formal services. It remains open to question *what* mechanisms rural families use to cope successfully with their changing environment.

The specific coping strategies used by rural families are probably not that radically different from those used by urban families. Some have argued that rural residents may enjoy some advantages when attempting to cope with crises. Bachrach (1981, p. 41), for example, has suggested that anecdotal accounts combined with limited empirical evidence would suggest that rural residents have "special and very important resources to tap." She characterized the following among the resources available: (a) the greater sense of community in rural areas; (b) rural tolerance of deviance; (c) better integrated and more easily reached natural helping networks in small towns and rural communities (refer to our earlier comments on this subject); and (d) the existence of indigenous human service extenders.

Despite the speculations, however, it is our conclusion that there is scant evidence to support the assertion that rural families are any more advantaged in their ability to cope with stress. Other factors—mutual respect, cohesiveness, family history, personal values, open patterns of communication and emotional stability—seem much more important than place of residence in predicting the ability to cope with stress. This is not to suggest that rural families have no resources to call upon in times of crisis. Indeed, research by Stinnett (1979), completed on a largely rural sample, demonstrated that many families have important, existing internal strengths that can be mobilized under appropriate circumstan-

ces. Ultimately, however, our ability to understand the coping mechanisms employed by rural families is limited by our lack of research on
the internal dynamics of these families (Coward & Smith, 1982).

We must not assume that similar events will result in comparable
amounts of stress or that urban and rural families will cope in the same
way. How the local culture interprets an event is an important factor in
determining not only coping strategies but also the final resolution of
stress by the family. For example, the lower prevalence of divorce in
rural communities, coupled with reported higher levels of disapproval
and social stigma, may persuade some people to continue low-quality
relationships (perhaps further escalating stress) or may provide even
more stress for those who separate despite the sanctions (Schumm &
Bollman, 1981). We can support or refute these speculations, however,
only after more research helps us to better understand the internal dynamics of rural families.

IMPLICATIONS FOR POLICY

In recent years both the numbers and the needs of rural families have
been all but ignored by legislators, bureaucrats, and news media. The
problems of the cities have grabbed public and political attention, and
cities get more than their share of tax dollars back in the form of grants,
loans, and special programs. Our values appear to be shaped by "me-
tropollyanna"—the delusion that sooner or later everyone will move to
the city and live happily ever after.

In addition to the domination of public attention by urban problems,
a second reason for the lack of rural-oriented policy is the myth that
"all is well in the country." The image of the rural family which we have
mentioned before in this chapter—the image of a life in bucolic sim-
plicity, surrounded by kin, church and benevolent county commission-
ers—has masked the real needs of rural people. There is no comprehensive
federal policy for rural America (Coward, 1980), and this neglect has
allowed many rural problems to "fall between the slats." How does this
urban bias in policymaking affect rural families under stress? One very
real way is in the social service delivery system. Some of the help these
families need could come from social service agencies, but their record
of service in rural areas is not very good.

One hindrance to service is the many clinical or counseling staff who
are urban-born and urban-educated. Unfamiliar with rural life, they
sometimes descend upon small towns like the proverbial

locust—insensitive to local customs and values and "hell bent" on sharing their professional wisdom with the native folks. Rural-oriented training programs for professionals in family medicine, psychology, social work, and gerontology have been developed and should improve the situation. Yet, the continued lack of delivery models reflecting a deep understanding of families in rural society and tailored to fit the needs of a particular community remains an obstacle. There has been some progress in designing uniquely rural systems but much more direct attention is needed before significant advances are won. A third obstacle is the obvious lack of a sound base of research data which can be used to guide the development and tailoring of social programs in rural communities. We need more information on a continuous basis about family life, the impact of social change and stressors on family relationships, and child and adult development in rural communities. We need a clearer picture of the impact of rural social service programs. We appear to be moving in this direction, but we have a long way to go. Coward (1981, pp. 18-19) expressed this shortcoming when he cautioned that the

> . . . changes that rural families experience occur in a psychosocial, or attitudinal, environment that is consistently different from urban society. Rural America is not simply a smaller scale urban setting. Rural America is qualitatively different and unique from metropolitan America. Because of those contextual differences, we must be cautious about assuming that the same general trend in families holds identical or even similar meanings in the two environments. The direction of change is important; but ultimately the impact of change on individuals and families will, in large part, be determined by the meaning attached by the community to the change.

LIFE SATISFACTION IN RURAL FAMILIES: A PARADOX

Despite the potential for stress that exists in rural families and their consistently disadvantaged status on major objective measures of the quality of life, rural residents repeatedly express greater happiness and satisfaction with their total lives than do urban family members (Tremblay, Walker, & Dillman, 1983). This seems to be a perplexing paradox. Tremblay et al. (1983) have argued that although rural residents are aware of the inadequacies and shortcomings of their communities, they simply give greater weight to other factors when assessing their overall life satisfaction.

Be cautious, however, in interpreting this information because, as a whole, Americans rate their life satisfaction high. "Rather than urban families being dissatisfied with their lives, they are just *less* satisfied when compared to rural families" (Tremblay et al., 1983, p. 21). Furthermore, reports of high life satisfaction do not mean that there is less stress, just as lower satisfaction should not be equated with the presence of stress. The two phenomena are different and their association or causal relationship is complex.

CONCLUSION

Contrary to popular belief, living in rural America is filled with the harsh realities of modern life. Rural residents share many of the problems faced by their urban counterparts, and some of these are even more prevalent in rural America or made worse by the rural context in which they occur.

A factor to be considered equally important in the country as it is in the city is change. Life in rural areas does not remain untouched in its alleged serenity; rather, it is equally pressured by the spirit of change. Larger farms, fewer farms, fewer people working on farms, greater off-farm employment, and the increased labor force participation of rural women constitute significant changes in rural life that have occurred over the years. Recent migration shifts back to rural areas add to the dilemma faced by an already large and stable rural population.

We suggest not only that stress is a part of contemporary life for rural families, but also that it may have a different impact because of the milieu and context in which it occurs. We recommend caution in accepting the bucolic perceptions and idyllic images of life in the country, for to do so is to add to the mythology that has already hampered efforts to provide adequate and effective services to rural families and their communities.

CHAPTER

14

Economic Stress: Family Financial Management

MARY ANN NOECKER GUADAGNO

Newlyweds, Charles, 27, and Valerie, 25, live in an apartment about one mile from where they work in a Northwest U.S. city. They are careful shoppers and have furnished their apartment with antiques and other assorted flea-market treasures. The Smiths own one car, a 1980 Chevy Citation, and receive low cost medical care at an HMO as part of their employee benefit package. They have opened charge accounts at two large department stores to establish a good credit rating. They plan to save about $1,000 this year, since to date neither has any savings. While they manage to pay present living expenses, repay student loans and wedding expenses, reserve funds for entertainment, and save a minimal amount, Valerie wonders if they will ever really be able to afford a home, children, and the boat they dream of—among other things. It is stressful simply attempting to make ends meet!

For the Smiths, inflation remains a major source of economic stress from the external environment. Although inflation is a historical, cyclical, economic phenomenon in America, it has only recently been examined by social scientists as a stressor or source of family stress (Caplovitz,

1979). Virtually no one since the Great Depression (Angell, 1936; Cavan & Ranck, 1938) has attempted to examine how and why some families are strengthened by severe economic conditions such as inflation, while other succumb to financial disaster. In the 1980s, Americans are experiencing high levels of unemployment and inflation, a phenomenon dubbed "stagflation" by economists (Juster, 1979; Robbins, Britton, Coats, Friedman, Jay, & Laidler, 1974; Solomon, 1975). This environmental stressor continues to affect family choice regarding allocation of income to consumption, savings, and investment. Families are forced to cope with the general economy by making adjustments within their own family microeconomy. Such adjustments may have profound effects on the quality of American life (Barrett & Driscoll, 1976; Caplovitz, 1979; Hollister & Palmer, 1972; Minarik, 1978).

This chapter will: 1) define inflation (the family stressor event)—what causes it, how it is measured, and how it affects family resources; 2) describe the types of families most affected by inflation, and 3) discuss family coping strategies used by families to deal with inflation.

DEFINING INFLATION

Inflation is a general term that refers to an increase in some weighted average of the prices of goods and services produced or consumed in an economy. More basically, inflation is a continuing increase in the general price level of goods and services. As prices increase, the value of money decreases. In family economic terms, the value of money is often described as family purchasing power or "real" dollars. For example, "double digit" inflation in 1980 caused the greatest decline in real median family income during the post World War II era, the first statistically significant decline since the 1974-75 recession. Median 1980 family income was $21,023, compared to $19,587 in 1979. However, adjusting for a 13.5% increase in 1980 consumer prices over 1979, real 1980 median family income declined by 5.5% (U. S. Bureau of the Census, 1981b).

Causes

There is no tidy, single theory to adequately explain what causes inflation. Different schools of economics subscribe to different theories. Two basic types of inflation are demand-pull and cost-push. Demand-pull inflation occurs when the supply of available money is greater than the available goods and services for sale. When family demand for certain goods and services is caused by an excessive increase in the quantity of money in circulation, prices tend to increase. This phenomenon is often typified by the phrase "too many dollars chasing too few goods." For example, excess demand from the Defense Department during the Vietnam War caused the first bouts with demand-pull inflation in the United States.

Inflation may also be of the cost-push type. Cost-push inflation occurs when increasing costs to produce goods and services, coupled with rising wages paid to employees, push prices upward (structural explanation). A cost-push inflation implies that inflation is caused by the power of large corporations and unions who are hypothetically free to raise their prices and wage rates at will.

Of course, many other phenomena may be contributing factors to inflation: government fiscal and monetary policies, employment levels, supply and demand in the markets, changes in foreign markets (e.g., the 1973-74 oil embargo and 1978-79 crisis in Iran), and expectations or consumer sentiment about inflation.

Measuring Inflation

There are various aggregate measures of inflation: the Consumer Price Index (CPI), Gross National Product (GNP), and the Wholesale Price Index. The CPI measures change in retail prices over time, for a specific combination or market basket of United States goods and services. Gross National Product (GNP) is a measure of total goods and services produced in the economy for a certain period of time. The Wholesale Price Index (WPI) measures change in wholesale prices over time for a specific combination of goods and services.

The most common measure used by families as an indicator of inflation is the Consumer Price Index (CPI). The CPI compares the cost of a current fixed market basket of goods and services to its cost at a previous time. Prices are compared to a base period (1967) index. For example, a given market basket indexed at 181.8 in 1977 could have been purchased for $100.00 in 1967 (CPI = 100), but would cost $181.80 in 1977 (U. S. Bureau of Labor Statistics, 1978). The CPI market basket is composed of a typical mix of goods and services purchased by an average American family. Market basket items are identified, selected, and updated by the U. S. Department of Labor based upon United States surveys of consumer preferences. Each item is weighted to reflect its relative importance in the total budget for the typical American family.

Until 1978, the CPI was based on Clerical and Wage Earners' Budgets. At present, the U. S. Department of Labor, Bureau of Labor Statistics publishes a revised CPI for all Urban Consumers (CPI-U), which covers approximately 80% of the total noninstitutional civilian population, and a revised CPI for Urban Wage Earners and Clerical Workers (CPI-W), representing about half of the population covered by CPI-U. CPI-U includes groups which have traditionally been excluded from the CPI, such as professionals, technicians, managers, self-employed individuals, short-term and unemployed workers, and retirees, in addition to urban wage earners and clerical workers (for details see U. S. Bureau of Labor Statistics, 1978, 1980a).

The CPI has its limitations as a measure of inflation for family use. First, the CPI reflects an average American's expenditures for goods and services. Consequently, there is no consideration of individual or regional preferences. Families who do not buy the same products or services need to be aware of which items are reflected in the average budget in order to estimate how their budget might differ. Second, families living in rural America are not included in the urban budget analysis. Third, the CPI is not a cost of living budget. It only illustrates how much prices have changed from a base year. It does not tell how much income is needed to live in any particular city or region in the United States. Fourth, the CPI reflects neither changes in family expenditure patterns nor adjustments to new services or products.

How Inflation Affects Family Resources

Since the poor spend a larger proportion of income on food, gasoline, and home heating fuels compared to affluent families, they experience greater increases in their living costs for these specific items during periods of inflation. For example, Table 1 shows that, in Autumn 1979, urban families at the lowest BLS budget group spent 31% of their income on food while those in the highest group spent about 21% (for details of family budgets see U. S. Bureau of Labor Statistics, 1980b). Thus, as food prices rose approximately 22.2% from 1978 to 1979, the financial burden fell more heavily on the poor (U. S. Bureau of Labor Statistics, 1980b).

In contrast, higher inflationary prices erode the value of fixed-value assets (e.g., furniture) and reduce the real value of debts. However, property such as the family home, which is not fixed in value, may even gain in value relative to the increase in consumer prices. Thus, upper-income families generally remain well-off during inflationary periods.

TABLE 1
Annual Budgets for a Four-Person Urban Family, at Three Levels of Living
Autumn 1979[a]

COMPONENT†	LOWER	%	INTERMEDIATE	%	HIGH	%
Total Budget	$12,585		$20,517		$30,317	
Total family consumption	10,234	81%	15,353	74%	21,069	70%
Food	3,911	31%	5,044	25%	6,360	21%
Housing	2,409	19%	4,594	22%	6,971	23%
Transportation	1,004	8%	1,851	9%	2,411	8%
Clothing	866	7%	1,235	6%	1,804	6%
Personal care	323	3%	433	2%	613	2%
Medical care	1,171	9%	1,176	6%	1,227	4%
Other family consumption	550	4%	1,021	5%	1,684	6%
Other items	539	4%	877	4%	1,478	5%
Social security and disability	781	6%	1,256	6%	1,413	5%
Personal income taxes	1,032	8%	3,031	15%	6,357	21%

Note: Because of rounding, sums of individual items may not equal totals.
†For details see: U.S. Bureau of Labor Statistics. *Handbook of Labor Statistics* (Bulletin 2070). Washington, DC: U.S. Government Printing Office, 1980, pp. 385-399.

The very poor are not likely to feel much effect in either direction, since they own neither assets nor debts. The impact on middle-class families is less certain. There is greater variability in this group concerning indebtedness and composition of asset portfolios.

In sum, inflation affects family resources as follows: (a) The poor experience greater increases in their living costs for food, gasoline, and home heating fuels, since the poor spend a larger proportion of their income for these items; (b) upper-income families may suffer from a decrease in the value of their fixed value assets; however, increases in the value of real-estate and reductions in the real value of debts generally help them to keep even or slightly ahead of inflation; and (c) the inflationary effects on the middle class remain variable, depending on types and amounts of assets owned and debts outstanding.

FAMILY TYPES AFFECTED BY INFLATION

When the cost of living rises and unemployment increases, many families suffer, but not all. What is the extent to which families are suffering? In general, we know that the U. S. poverty threshold for a nonfarm family of four was $8,414 in 1980 (U. S. Bureau of the Census, 1981b). U. S. Census Bureau data show that, in 1980, the number of poor increased by 3.2 million persons, for a total of 29.3 million or approximately 13% of the United States population (U. S. Bureau of the Census, 1981b).

Most segments of the United States population were affected by the increase in poverty between 1979 and 1980. Table 2 shows that those hardest hit by inflation were Blacks and Spanish-speaking people, those under age 65, children under 18 years in poor families, farm families, central city residents in metropolitan areas, families living in the South, families with a female householder—no husband present, and married couple families and females living alone. Thus, as would be expected, assuming there is some variation in effect by location, factors affecting the impact of inflation on family income and consumption are: race, age, family size, occupation, and family type. In general, as income increases, the impact of inflation decreases; Blacks and Spanish-speaking individuals are harder hit by inflation than whites; those under age 65 are worse off then those over 65; as family size increases, the impact of inflation increases; farm families are harder hit by inflation than nonfarm families; and single women or households headed by women fare worse than their male counterparts.

TABLE 2. Persons, Families, and Unrelated Individuals Below the Poverty Level in 1979 and 1980[a] (Numbers in Thousands. Persons, Families, and Unrelated Individuals as of March of the Following Year)

SELECTED CHARACTERISTICS	BELOW POVERTY LEVEL			POVERTY RATE		
	1980	1979	Difference	1980	1979	Difference
All persons	29,272	26,072	*3,200	13.0	11.7	*1.2
White	19,699	17,214	*2,485	10.2	9.0	*1.2
Black	8,579	8,050	*529	32.5	31.0	**1.5
Spanish origin[b]	3,491	2,921	*570	25.7	21.8	*3.9
Under 65 years	25,401	22,390	*3,011	12.7	11.3	*1.4
65 years and over	3,871	3,682	**189	15.7	15.2	0.5
Related children under 18 years	11,359	10,193	*1,166	18.1	16.2	*1.9
Nonfarm	28,282	25,279	*3,003	12.9	11.7	*1.2
Farm	990	793	**197	17.5	13.3	*4.2
In metropolitan areas	18,021	16,134	*1,887	11.9	10.7	*1.2
In central cities	10,644	9,720	*924	17.2	15.7	1.5
Outside central cities	7,377	6,415	*962	8.2	7.2	*1.0
Outside metropolitan areas	11,251	9,937	*1,314	15.4	13.8	*1.6
North and West	16,919	14,974	*1,945	11.3	10.1	*1.2
South	12,353	11,098	*1,255	16.5	15.0	*1.5
All families	6,217	5,461	*756	10.3	9.2	*1.1
Married couple families	3,032	2,640	*392	6.2	5.4	*0.8
Male householder, no wife present	213	176	**37	11.0	10.2	0.8
Female householder, no husband present	2,972	2,645	*327	32.7	30.4	*2.3
All unrelated individuals	6,227	5,743	*484	22.9	21.9	*1.0
Male	2,109	1,972	**137	17.4	16.9	0.5
Female	4,118	3,771	*347	27.4	26.0	*1.4

*Significant at the 95% confidence level.
**Significant between the 90% and 95% confidence levels.
[a]For details see: U.S. Bureau of the Census, 1981b.
[b]Persons of Spanish origin may be of any race.

In sum, data show that the upper and middle classes are not as affected by inflation as are the classes below them. Families most vulnerable to the inflationary crunch tend to be poor, Black or Spanish-speaking, under age 65, large (over four persons), those whose breadwinners have relatively low occupational prestige, those who live on farms, and those headed by women. The single most important factor explaining the inflation crunch is amount of income.

Extent to Which Families are Suffering

In the study of family stress, stress is conceptualized as the distressed family's unmanaged response (tension) to a stressor (Hill, 1949). The extent to which families are suffering in inflation can be defined as the felt discrepancy between their income and rising prices. A major concern of family economists is: "How are families in the same objective circumstances, e.g., income, education, occupation level, etc., responding to inflation?"

Data from the Great Depression (Angell, 1936; Bakke, 1940, 1942; Cavan & Ranck, 1938; Komarovsky, 1940; Zawadski & Lazarsfeld, 1935) and historical reviews (Bennett & Elder, 1979; Moen, Kain, & Elder, 1981; Westin, 1976) provide insight about the extent to which families suffer due to economic deprivation as a function of temporary or relative income loss to family purchasing power (in contrast to more permanent or chronic poverty).

Elder (1981) concluded that in the 1930s family suffering due to economically induced stress varied depending upon differential exposure to and severity of the economic loss. Severity was defined as a function of the duration and extent of income loss. An economic loss of up to 20-30% of real 1929 family income in 1932 did not appear to constitute genuine hardship. However, marked deprivation resulted in families as income loss approached 40%.

Limited opportunities for advanced education and consequently limited economic means dictated a lifestyle of denial and postponement of material goods acquisition for many. Family adaptation to economic hardship led to a reorganization of family roles and responsibilities within the household sector. During the 1930s a majority of women worked outside the home to supplement family income. Yet the working mother maintained a central role in family activities, especially if her husband was unemployed.

The eldest daughter often played a major role in managing the household. Sons tended to work in paid employment outside the home. As a result, young men from economically deprived families experienced an accelerated push toward social and economic independence. Moreover, they reported placing high value on marital stability, family life, job security, adequate income, and fewer children than the noneconomically deprived group. Following marriage, young women tended to opt for both career and family. Since a majority of their mothers had worked outside the home, employment was viewed as an extension of the wife-mother role.

The greater the gap between pre- and post-Depression family income or level of living, the greater families suffered as they attempted to lower standards and give up symbols of family status. The effect of income loss was moderated by the degree of occupational skill of family members, past experiences with unemployment or economic loss, availability of credit, amount of savings and investments, family size, extent of mutual family activities, rigidity of family roles, flexibility of family standards, and availability of social support networks (Bakke, 1940). Despite major shifts in family roles, responsibilities, and resources, few incidences of marital discontent were reported.

More recently, Caplovitz (1979) presented respondents with a series of statements (with which they could agree or disagree) that tapped their experiences with inflation and the degree to which they were hurting. The most widely accepted statements, endorsed by at least half of the sample were: a) Inflation is depressing; b) money is becoming worthless; c) luxury items are excluded from the family budget; and d) items are repaired rather than thrown away. Results showed that 67% of the families perceived inflationary stress as medium to very high.

Caplovitz (1979) found that the more families felt they suffered from inflation, the more they reported that their marriages suffered. Furthermore, as the incidence of staying at home increased, due in part to cutbacks in family entertainment, reports of marital strain increased. Other correlates of marital strain in inflation were family size and employment status. The larger the family, the greater the incidence of marital strain. Reports of marital strain were higher for the unemployed than for the employed.

Caplovitz found that in some families economic pressures resulted in closer ties between spouses as they increased communication to cope with economic adversity. Parents reported that even children were more helpful and attempted to pitch in more frequently than when the family was not faced with economic hardship.

COPING WITH INFLATION

How can families cope with inflation? What can families do to deal effectively with prevalent, stressful, economic conditions?

Hill (1949), Deacon and Firebaugh (1981), and Burr (1973) all emphasize the importance of family resources availability and perceived availability in explaining how severe the family's reaction to a stressful event will be. The primary hardship related to the stress of inflation is the loss of family purchasing power. McCubbin, Joy, Cauble, Comeau, Patterson, and Needle (1980) identified personal resources (e.g., economic well-being, education, health, and personality), social supports (e.g., emotional esteem, network), and family system resources (e.g., family adaptability and cohesion) as the chief resources studied in relation to stress.

The process of coping with inflation involves *cognitive coping strategies* such as individual and family acceptance of the fact that they are no longer living in a time of plenty. Financial expectations for single family dwellings, two cars, or educating children may no longer be realistic. Choices and substitutions will have to be made among competing scarce resources.

This chapter focuses on the stressor, inflation, as an economic condition which levies constraints on the family's choice of goods and services. Coping is explained within the context of a *family management* framework. Management is defined as planning and implementing family resources to meet family demands, i.e., goals and events requiring action (Deacon & Firebaugh, 1981, p. 29). Deacon and Firebaugh (1981) maintain that family resources are human (e.g., personal, family) and material (e.g., income, assets).

Personal Resources

Literature on personal resources used to manage in inflation is scant. Referring to George's (1980) four basic components of personal resources—economic well-being, education, health, and personality characteristics—we can surmise that there might well be some changes in an individual's stock of personal resources as a direct or indirect result of inflation. For example, as family members are affected by inflation, their sense of economic well-being may decrease, education may have to be postponed due to increases in tuition and shrinking family purchasing power, health could deteriorate if adequate health care is no longer affordable, and personalities may change as individuals become more frugal.

Research on family coping in the Great Depression (Angell, 1936; Cavan & Ranck, 1938) illustrated that family response to economic stress may be positive (e.g., families may grow stronger as they grow closer to combat inflation) or negative (e.g., family stability may be badly shaken as families struggle to maintain their accustomed standard of living, ambitions, and aspirations).

A few investigators have examined emotional, esteem, and network support, i.e., social supports, as a function of providing money, gifts, loans, or other financial assistance in emergencies (Granovetter, 1973; Lee, 1979; Troll, 1971). To date, little research has attended to the question of what role money plays in how effectively families cope with stress.

Material Resources

The importance of using a management framework to manage family financial resources has been illustrated by Deacon and Firebaugh (1981) and Guadagno (1981). A majority of families rely on earned income as their chief financial resource. As previously stated, 1980 median family income was $21,023, up 7.3% from 1979 median income, but down 5.5% in real median family income (see Table 3). This decline in family purchasing power and consequent decline in family living levels will mandate psychological, social, and behavioral adjustments. Assuming that personal, social, and psychological resource adjustments are necessary, the following section will discuss potential managerial adjustment strategies specifically related to family income, production, and consumption behavior.

Managerial Strategies

Families can adapt by using any one or a combination of four managerial strategies. They may attempt to: (a) increase income; (b) reduce expenses; (c) extend resources on hand by learning new skills for self-sufficiency; or (d) substitute, exchange, or share goods and services among family and friends instead of purchasing new items. These options are not feasible for all individuals or family types. Low-income families or those living on fixed incomes, for example, already have limited resources and consequently limited options for coping with in-

TABLE 3
Median Family Income in 1979 and 1980 in Current and Constant
Dollars, by Selected Characteristics[a]

		MEDIAN FAMILY INCOME		
			1979	Percent Change in Real Income
SELECTED CHARACTERISTICS	1980	Constant Dollars	Current Dollars	
All families	$21,023	$22,236	$19,587	* −5.5
Race and Spanish Origin				
White	21,904	23,203	20,439	* −5.6
Black	12,674	13,139	11,574	** −3.5
Spanish origin[b]	14,717	16,085	14,169	* −8.5
Type of residence				
Nonfarm	21,151	22,339	19,678	* −5.3
Farm	15,755	18,483	16,281	* −14.8
Inside metropolitan areas	22,590	23,848	21,007	* −5.3
Outside metropolitan areas	18,069	19,190	16,904	* −5.8
Region				
Northeast	21,856	23,411	20,622	* −6.6
North Central	21,736	23,353	20,571	* −6.9
South	19,142	19,923	17,550	* −3.9
West	22,281	23,487	20,689	* −5.1

*Significant at the 95% confidence level.
**Significant between the 90% and 95% confidence levels.
[a]For details see: U.S. Bureau of the Census, 1981b.
[b]Persons of Spanish origin may be of any race.

flation. Government intervention will remain vital to ensure a minimal level of living for these families.

Increasing Family Income. One obvious way to maintain the family's level of living during inflation is to increase family income. Normal channels of increasing income via job promotion or salary increases are often inadequate or impossible during periods of high inflation. Thus, families may opt to: allow the chief wage earner to take a second job or work overtime, send another family member into the labor force (typically the wife), or engage in illegal activity in order to increase their income. Caplovitz (1979) found in an urban sample that 28% of chief wage earners worked overtime, 16% reported an additional family member had entered the labor force, 4% held two jobs, and 10% engaged in "off the books" or illegal activities such as collecting unemployment insurance while working or working without reporting income for tax purposes.

Working overtime appears to be a major coping strategy to increase income in inflation, a viable option for both singles and married family members. The opportunity to work overtime is occupation specific, however. Thus, blue and white collar workers are more likely to use this strategy than professionals or farmers.

The increasing incidence of wives joining the labor force has been well documented (Johnson, 1979; U. S. Bureau of Labor Statistics, 1980c). Recent growth in the female labor force has resulted primarily from increased numbers of working married women with young children (U.S. Bureau of the Census, 1981b). Data suggest more permanent labor force participation by women; economic necessity remains the primary motivator for female labor force attachment.

Although in the past a second job might have helped families in inflation, the present high rate of unemployment presents a major structural barrier to this alternative. Although individuals and family members may be willing to work a second job, many cannot find one. Single parents, young families with preschool children, semi-skilled or unskilled workers, and minorities are most likely to be affected by job scarcity.

Decreasing Family Expenditures. Reducing family consumption expenditures is a second strategy families can use to cope with inflation. Typically, families dispense with luxuries first, then essentials. In order of importance, families tend to reduce expenditures for meals at home, entertainment, eating out, and clothing (Caplovitz, 1979).

Food expenditures may be cut by shifting to less expensive goods, using shopping lists, planning weekly menus around advertised specials, comparing prices, and buying in bulk. Although home gardening, canning, and freezing may help reduce food expenditures, families must carefully examine the time versus cost trade-offs, as well as initial outlays for equipment and maintenance. For example, it may be less expensive for a working mother to purchase canned and frozen vegetables on sale than to invest her time and energy into gardening and purchasing a freezer or canning equipment.

Entertainment appears to be the second major category where families cut back. As families seek less expensive leisure activities, they may increase use of community resources such as parks, libraries, and museums, take vacations closer to home, exchange homes for vacationing, engage in more family games, and share babysitting arrangements more frequently.

Clothing outlays can be reduced by doing without new clothes, shifting to less expensive clothing, shopping factory outlets, eliminating dry-cleanables, redesigning old clothing, or sharing clothing with friends and relatives. Although home sewing is a viable option to reduce expenses, as with home production of food, time versus cost trade-offs must be accurately and realistically assessed.

Despite rapidly rising fuel prices, families have been reluctant to cut back on transportation. Alternatives to the two-car family include car pooling or increased use of public transportation. When purchasing a new automobile, families can reduce future fuel costs by selecting a car with a smaller engine. Consumer information sources such as *Consumer Reports* (published by Consumers' Union) provide families with accurate, timely guides to major family purchases. The cost of credit for new car purchases can be reduced by using the shortest repayment schedule with a large down payment. Vehicle costs can be kept to a minimum by careful choice of repair shops and insuring only major risks. Cost of air travel can be minimized by purchasing tickets at special rates when reservations are made in advance.

Adjusting consumption patterns with emphasis on reducing demand for energy—gas, fuel oil, electricity—is vital and will become increasingly important in the near future. For many, this adjustment will not be easy. Smaller, energy tight homes, less home heat and air-conditioning, fewer electrical kitchen and bathroom appliances, and less frequent appliance usage could result in considerable financial savings.

Extending Resources on Hand. Extending resources on hand involves attempts to increase efficiency or self-reliance. This coping strategy may be one of the most realistic for a majority of American families. Increasing efficiency of resource use includes reducing waste and repairing or redesigning rather than discarding. Increased reliance on friends for help with babysitting, lending money, exchanging clothes, sharing transportation and food can help extend resources.

Substitution, Exchange, or Sharing. A fourth strategy for coping with the ravages of inflation is to substitute handmade gifts or to exchange or share goods and services among family and friends rather than insisting on new purchases.

Dysfunctional Coping Methods

Ironically, the process of making family income and consumption adaptations to cope with inflation may create family tension. As the double ABCX model (see Chapter 1) predicts, the coping strategy may itself be a stressor. Conversely, if adjustments are not made, family conflict may occur. For instance, conflict may arise over a parental decision not to replace a teenager's television set. Since the teenager is accustomed to the privacy and convenience of having his or her own television set, shared use of the family television may not be easy. Roskies and Lazarus (1980) have documented this phenomenon and concluded that it is possible for a family member to make a change in the use of family resources that can actually create more tension within the system.

One cannot simply conclude, however, that stress resulting from additional demands placed on the family in inflationary economic conditions will lead to child abuse, divorce, separation, drug or alcohol abuse, crime, bankruptcy, extended use of credit, murder, suicide, insanity, or illness. Studies of response to a variety of stressful events show that it is not the stressor *per se* that leads to family dysfunction or breakdown, but the absence or presence of explanations which help the family understand what happened or is happening and how it can rearrange its immediate environment to overcome the inopportune situation. In other words, it is the family's *perception* of the event (the cC factor in the double ABCX model) which determines how much stress will be experienced.

Specific dysfunctional coping methods individuals or families might employ to deal with inflationary related stress are:

(a) mismanaging finances, e.g., overspending or making unwise investments;

(b) increasing income at the expense of straining family relationships;

(c) decreasing expenses to the point of neglecting provisions for adequate protection against personal economic risks, e.g., property losses, illness, premature retirement or death;

(d) increasing self-sufficiency at the expense of personal or family social development;

(e) relying on social, governmental or other social and financial support programs rather than developing personal resources and skills to earn an adequate income in the labor force; and

(f) failure to adjust economic aspirations for a realistic family income, living level, and perhaps even number of children in light of increasing resource shortages.

PROFESSIONAL ASSISTANCE FOR THE FINANCIALLY DISTRESSED

Programs of prevention seem more desirable than programs of intervention, although both can be effective and are presently employed by professionals and clinicians to help individuals and families cope with inflation.

Preventative educational and counseling programs are infrequently provided, often on an informal or selective basis. Several commercial banks, for instance, provide financial planning assistance free of charge to customers with sizable accounts. Financial consultants, educators, or counselors may present formal university courses, noncredit courses taught at a convenient location in the community, or a mini-series of lectures to interested family members. Obviously, families or family members self select into such programs. Consequently, it has been difficult to standardize substantive programs of prevention for families.

Intervention programs for financial distress are by far the norm. Wage-Earner Plans, commonly referred to as "Chapter 13 plans," offer a less severe way than bankruptcy for families to cope with a failure to pay bills. Under such plans, a plan is developed and approved by the court, thus enabling a family to repay debts in a reasonable amount of time and with reasonable routine payments. In some cases, portions of the original debt are actually dissolved by the court. In regular bankruptcy, the court liquidates a majority of family assets and sells them to repay creditors. Families are left with the barest essentials and a ruined credit rating.

Consolidation loan programs may be an effective method of coping with financial stress if the family can refrain from any further use of credit. Consolidation loans are offered by commercial banks who merge all outstanding debts into one payment and spread payments out over a longer period of time. The advantages of this program may be overweighed by typical high interest rates charged for this service.

Consumer Credit Counseling is a nonprofit organization offered throughout the country to help families in financial trouble by assisting them to set up a realistic family budget and deal with creditors.

Although such programs may actually reduce family debt caused in part by the financial ravages of inflation, they are often unguided by any systematic treatment modality that could effectively change family dysfunction and help family members to reevaluate attitudes about economic well-being or plan and implement controlling attitudes and behaviors that reinforce and facilitate family adaptation to the stressor of inflation.

CONCLUSIONS AND IMPLICATIONS FOR POLICY AND RESEARCH

At a practical level, there is a vital need for additional consumer education programs at the high school, university, and community programming level to teach families how to manage resources more effectively in light of current inflationary pressures. Indeed, if families understand inflation, its causes and consequences, they will be more psychologically prepared to cope with inflation in an effective way. Several timely and practical prescriptions have been offered throughout this chapter to help families deal with this stressor, e.g., avoid using credit, invest in a home, use shopping lists. The list is endless and families will adapt those they find consistent with family values, goals, and resource levels.

A need exists for more systematic and rigorous research to provide information about how families cope with inflation. Researchers and clinicians will first need to identify measures of objective and subjective family economic stress, and the extent to which families perceive and objectively experience stress as a function of inflation at different life cycle stages, at different income levels, and at critical life events such as divorce, death, and separation. Second, we need to identify which coping strategies are most and least effective for dealing with inflation, why, and in what types of families they are used. Third, we need to identify family managerial patterns (e.g., goal setting, planning and controlling attitudes and behaviors) that facilitate family adaptation to chronic inflation.

In sum, family adaptation might be enhanced by educational programs geared at consumer awareness, self-help skills, value clarification, resource management, and an understanding of family dynamics. Counseling programs of prevention rather than intervention will allow families to more effectively and easily adapt to the stressor event—inflation. Coping with inflationary economic pressures will remain a major challenge for families and family members in the 1980s.

15

Bridging Normative and Catastrophic Family Stress

HAMILTON I. McCUBBIN
and CHARLES R. FIGLEY

Frank and Ann Leonard, a Black family in Ohio, have done well for themselves and their two children (Jeff, age 16, and Jennifer, age nine). They own their own home and live in a nice community. However, during the past three months, they have faced several transitions: Ann's mother died unexpectedly, her father became ill soon after, and during this period Ann returned to work fulltime as a nurse. Ann really wanted to return to her career and knew that the family budget would also be helped by this decision. When asked by a casual acquaintance how the family is doing, the Leonards are quick to reply that "everything is fine." But is it?

Recently Frank Leonard asked his friend, Todd, for some advice. Frank has been feeling depressed and expressed concern about his marriage, which seemed to be "going downhill." He blames his mother-in-law's death for this, since Ann and her mother were very close and Ann can't seem to adjust. Todd would like to help Frank, but is not sure what to focus upon (Ann's mother's death, her father's illness, her return to work). Frank's resentment at having to pick up some of the home management and child-care and Ann's higher salary are other possible stressors.

The Leonard family is in transition and in crisis. Like most families faced with normative transitions (grandparent's death, shifts in employment), the Leonards struggle with a host of pressures and demands which appear to occur at the same time. The expectation that they "ought" to be able to handle these "normal" occurrences exacerbates the tension.

NORMATIVE TRANSITIONS AND CATASTROPHES

The chapters presented in this first volume of *Stress and the Family* have attempted to describe and provide some understanding of families like the Leonards and their characteristic behaviors in response to one class of stressors: normative transitions. These chapters, we hope, shed some light upon the dynamic and complex manner in which stressors and coping reactions curtail family functioning or, conversely, promote family development and adaptation. They call our attention to normative transitions and accompanying stress as important areas for future research, intervention, and policy formation.

Every chapter in this book emphasizes the critical importance of resources within and outside the family as a component of family coping. These resources—be they tangible or intangible, formal or informal, general or specific, free or expensive, accessible or inaccessible—must be identified and the distribution equitably established in anticipation of need.

The Leonard family, for example, depended on the community for resources related to the death of a parent/grandparent, or Ann's skills of nursing, and on the emotional support of a friend. Because such critical times are infrequent, they do not place undue strain on extant resources. Because they are more or less common life occurrences, the family had some idea of the most appropriate ways of managing the situation and could draw on the advice of its social support network.

Thus, families generally operate on a predictable, normal cycle, anticipating and accepting a sequence of events that will occur throughout the life course. These predictable transitions may, however, be disrupted by unanticipated or traumatic events. The family rhythm and routine may be disrupted significantly by anticipated life events coming at unanticipated times—"off schedule." The death of a parent, for example, during the child's school-age years rather than during his/her adulthood, teenage marriages, early retirement, or "late" childbearing may be considered off schedule. The timing of life and family transitions can become a major source of family stress and strain, since mobilizing sufficient resources may detract attention from other areas.

These observations clearly indicate that children change, adults change, and families change with different timetables through the life cycle. These internal transitions are influenced by cultural variation, environmental conditions, and social changes. These normative processes of change and transition predictably have a profound impact upon family vulnerability to nonnormative stressors occurring concurrently and upon the family's ability to recover from such disruptions.

But what about situations which neither family members nor any of their social network have ever anticipated or experienced? What about situations that so suddenly and completely overwhelm family members that their entire lives are disrupted? What about situations which are so traumatic to one of the family members that merely discussing the trauma-related events produces nightmares, flashbacks, depression, and terror? In these situations the family rarely can rely on past experiences and the guidance of others and is left, at least for a time, to fend for itself. These families of catastrophe are the focus of Volume II of this series on *Stress and the Family*.

What Constitutes a Catastrophe?

In Volume II, Figley (Chapter 1) notes that a catastrophe is a classification of events which are associated with a wide gamut of stress-related consequences affecting the individuals who survive them and those the survivor turns to for comfort. Specifically, catastrophic stress is defined as "sudden and extreme threat to survival which is associated with a sense of helplessness, disruption, destruction, and loss." There is a wide range of events known to induce catastrophic stress, e.g., rape, war, terroristic captivity, and natural disasters.

The Importance of Family Support

Throughout the literature (e.g., Janis, 1971; Janis & Leventhal, 1968), it is clear that a primary antidote to both experiencing the catastrophe and adjusting to its memories is human contact, social support, and especially family support. But what if the entire family is affected simultaneously?

The families who experience catastrophic stress when members are together—the Ruskin family of Pendleton, Indiana whose home was completely destroyed by a tornado as they huddled together in the basement, for example—are at one end of a continuum. On the other end are families experiencing catastrophic stress *through* the experiences conveyed to them by a family member after surviving a catastrophic event (e.g., a daughter returning from college and telling her parents that she was raped the previous week). In the latter case the extent to which family members (a) care about and empathize with the victim, (b) perceive the victim's experiences as catastrophic (i.e., sudden and extreme threat), and (c) sense that the victimized family member is recovered or recovering is associated with the level of catastrophic stress.

The 1979-1981 Iran hostage crisis in which over 50 Americans were held hostage in that country provides an illustration of the impact on the family of a catastrophic event. At no time were any family members of these hostages in any danger, yet, according to recent research, many experienced classic signs of catastrophic stress disorders: depression, anxiety, dramatic mood shifts, sleep disruption, social isolation, paranoia, difficulty concentrating, excessive anger and hostility, guilt, and various phobias associated with forms of telecommunication (which may bring word of the status of their hostaged family member) (Burgess & Baldwin, 1981; Figley, 1980, 1981, 1982).

Reports, as yet unpublished, reveal that even 18 months after the return of the family member, loved ones still have occasional nightmares and experience other traumatic reactions linked with the experience. Added to the real danger to the hostages and the concomitant anxiety of the families were the extreme disruptions in the lifestyle, routine, and image of the family. Prior to November 1979, these families were coping with the normative and transitional stressors of life as best they could. Suddenly one of their members was caught in a dangerous situation which he or she may not have survived. And because it was an event of national and international importance, soon the entire world was aware of them and the struggles they faced. This led to not only the stressor of danger to a family member but also the stressors of public recognition and attention—in sharp contrast to a lifestyle the families were used to.

THE RELATIONSHIP BETWEEN NORMATIVE
AND CATASTROPHIC STRESSORS

Stress is stress. At a biophysiological level, reactions to stress are the same, regardless of the source. However, in these volumes we have made a distinction between normative and catastrophic stressors. Family stress research emerged from an interest in family perceptions of and coping with crisis situations. According to Hill (1958, p. 139), families experience crisis as a "sharp or decisive change for which old or ongoing roles are inadequate" and, according to Burr (1973, p. 201), the "change has brought about disruption in the family system." Role inadequacy and disruption not withstanding, our emphasis in the series is less on crisis than on stressors and how families conceptualize and manage them.

Variations in Stressors

Thus far we have noted that, although family stress is generic, in that the signs and symptoms it causes (e.g., elevations in tension, arguments, fighting, drug use, sleeplessness, psychosomatic problems) are similar, the *sources* of stress can be classified in several ways. For example, stressors could be associated with particular family structures (e.g., stepfamilies, single parenthood, dual-career families), or with the stages of the life cycle (e.g., families with teenage children). Stressors may be classified as to whether they emerge primarily from inside the family (e.g., normative transitions discussed in Part I of this volume) or from outside (e.g., environmental stressors discussed in Part II of this volume). As a way of reviewing the special nature of normative transitional/ environmental stressors discussed in this volume and introducing the reader to the catastrophic stressors to be discussed in Volume II, we have constructed Table 1 to demonstrate yet another way of classifying stressors.

In reviewing the list of characteristics associated with family stressors, it should be obvious that the differences between normative and catastrophic stressors are on a continuum. In other words, the differences in reactions in two families whose primary income earner becomes unemployed, for example, depend on many factors; in the end, one family may experience this as a crisis, while the other is able to readjust with minimal disruption.

Time to Prepare. Normative family transitions, such as the birth of the first child, though stressful at the time, are often discussed well in advance, either explicitly or implicitly. As Miller and Myers-Walls (Chapter 4) note, couples rearrange their lives—both physically and emotionally—during the months prior to the birth. In contrast catastrophic stressors allow little or no time to prepare. The onset is sudden, with little or no warning, such as a tornado or the phone call in the middle of the night informing the parents that their son is being held hostage. There is no time to prepare. An immediate response is required.

Degree of Anticipation. Similarly, catastrophic events most often occur without any anticipation, thus preventing the family from planning and rehearsing a survival strategy. In contrast, normative family transitions are anticipated. Parents recall (though never in sufficient detail) their own adolescence and their struggles with their parents for independence and freedom. As a result, parents anticipate a certain level of conflict with their teenagers over dress, friends, dating behavior, and curfew hours.

Previous Experience. As parents become accustomed to the rollercoaster of emotions in their teenagers, they experience less stress (cf., Kidwell et al., Chapter 5). Parenting, some have suggested, is learning by doing, trial and error. Thus, previous experience is quite important to managing the stressors of life in general and parenthood in particular. In contrast, most catastrophes happen only once. Indeed, the degree to which ca-

TABLE 1

General Variations Between Normative and Catastrophic Stressors

Characteristics	NORMATIVE	CATASTROPHIC
Time to prepare	Some	Little to none
Degree of anticipation	Great	None
Previous experience	Some	None
Sources of Guidance	Many	Few, if any
Experienced by others	Universally	Infrequently
Time in "crisis"	None or little	Little to much
Sense of control	Moderate to high	Little to none
Sense of helplessness	Little to none	Moderate to high
Sense of loss	Some	Much
Sense of disruption	Some	Much
Sense of destruction	Some	Much
Degree of dangerousness	None	Much
Associated emotional problems	Some	Many
Associated medical problems	Some	Many

tastrophes are stressful is associated with the uniqueness of the experience (Figley, 1982). For the rape victim, for example, there are few if any experiences to draw upon for guidance and strength; the same is true for her family. Indeed, in these times a supportive friend's previous experiences in being victimized may be a key factor in both establishing rapport and helping the victim work through her experience (cf., Burge, Volume II, Chapter 7).

Sources of Guidance. Everyone is an expert on the family; only a few are experts on a catastrophe. Thus, parents may find that in times of normative transiton, such as the young child learning to use a toilet, that there are *too many* sources of guidance (e.g., neighbors, family physicians, books, child specialists) and they must choose the method of training that best suits them. If a parent of young children dies, however, the sources of guidance are few, if any, until the family can make contact with proper community (and at times kinship) resources for assistance (cf., Zuengler & Neubeck, Chapter 3, and Crosby & Jose, Volume II, Chapter 5).

Experienced by Others. The fact that many others have experienced normative life transitions helps in coping, since families feel they are not unique or alone in their struggles. In social gatherings it is an appropriate topic of conversation to speak of stressors of everyday family life—everyone has something to contribute. But as Hunter (Volume II, Chapter 10) points out, families of those held hostage or as prisoners of war believe that few if any know of their stress; they feel estranged from their neighbors and friends following, and especially during, captivity. Families of catastrophe are a small and elite club who are members not by choice but by circumstance. The key to coping often involves allowing them to talk with families in similar circumstances, just as parents experience reassurance in sharing experiences with other parents.

Time in "Crisis." If crisis is synonymous with disruption, as has been suggested (Burr, 1973), few normative family transitions last long as a crisis, though collectively (i.e., pile-up effect) they may prolong this crisis period. Mrs. Leonard's returning to work, for example, was exacerbated by the death of her mother and illness of her father, thus prolonging, perhaps, the disruption that would normally be part of a wife-mother's returning to work. When catastrophe strikes—such as a tornado suddenly destroying part of the Leonard's home—the crisis is not only sudden, but is often "disruptive" for quite some time.

Sense of Control and Helplessness. Just as individuals sense a loss of control and feel totally helpless part or much of the time during and following a catastrophe, families experience these things collectively. If the Leonards' home were hit by a tornado, the research on family reactions to disasters would predict (c.f., Smith, Volume II, Chapter 8) that they would feel powerless against the capricious actions of nature, unable to control their fate and the unfolding destruction; they would feel that their choices—especially during the storm—were severely limited. And after the destruction they might still feel out of control and helpless due to the conditions of their neighbors, community, and relief efforts. In contrast, families dealing with normative family transitions rarely feel out of control and helpless, though they certainly may feel that their options are severely restricted.

Sense of Disruption and Destruction. Normative family transitions are disruptive and bring certain new roles, responsibilities, rules, and routines. Fundamental changes in the marital relationship, for example, have been traced to the transition to parenthood (Figley, 1973). But, as illustrated by the hypothetical tornado noted above, catastrophes often leave deep and permanent changes: Significant disruption and destruction of a family's entire lifestyle may occur.

Degree of Danger. Perhaps the most significant difference between the two categories of stressors is the degree of danger to one or more family members. The threat of physical harm or death provokes the most intense human reactions and leaves an emotional imprint which often lasts a lifetime (Lifton, 1979). Thus, families are emotionally shaken by the oldest son's involvement in a near fatal auto accident, or a father's being held as a hostage by a bank robber, or the baby's being diagnosed as having an incurable, crippling disease.

Emotional Problems. It is clear that everyday family transitions are stressful and may cause considerable emotional reaction. In some cases, these emotional reactions become major problems which impair one or more family members. However, problems associated with transitional family stressors are rarely chronic.* A growing body of scientific literature cited in Volume II notes both the acute and chronic emotional

---

*This proposition, of course, is in conflict with psychoanalytic theory which posits that it is precisely stressful normative transitions within the family which account for adult and child emotional disturbance.

fallout from catastrophes: psychosomatic medical problems (noted below), sleep disorders, social isolation and conflict, depression, distorted perceptions of self and others, phobia, paranoia, sexual dysfunction, and other potentially impairing reactions.

Medical Problems. The stress-biophysiology connection has been confirmed by Selye (1956; 1974) and others (Ursin, Baade, & Levine, 1978). More specifically, researchers have attempted to quantify the medical risks of certain types of catastrophes (Dohrenwend & Dohrenwend, 1974). According to one group of researchers (Holmes & Rahe, 1967), for example, the highest health risk is the death of a spouse. Thus, stress leaves an unmistakable imprint on the people affected. Headaches are, perhaps, the most frequently experienced stress-related medical problem. And although a greater proportion of families of catastrophe experience these medical stress-related problems (e.g., hypertension, heart disease, asthma, skin disorders, influenza), these problems are also associated with the stress of normative life transitions.

Similarities in Coping

It should be clear from reading this volume that stress is an integral part of family life, while catastrophes force families to make immediate adjustments. Functional methods of coping with both normative and catastrophic stress are often universal and transcend all types and categories of stressors. Table 2 provides an inventory of these universal or generic coping characteristics.

After some discussion, Frank and Ann Leonard realized that the stressful events they were experiencing were creating some problems for the family, and they tried to find ways that would help to ease the strain. For example, they made a special effort to spend Sundays with Jeff and Jennifer, in some way the kids would really enjoy—going to a baseball game or having a picnic by a lake. Once during those months, Frank and Ann got away while the kids stayed with friends; it gave them a chance to relax, and to talk about some of their problems. The Leonards were able to (a) see their accumulating stressors in proper perspective (clarify and accept stressors); (b) view the situation as a family problem that everyone must adjust to (family-centered); and (c) solve (solution-oriented), while (d) showing high tolerance, commitment, and affection to other family members; (e) utilizing open channels of communication; (f) striving for high family cohesion; (g) maintaining appropriate family roles which are flexible and able to shift to meet family needs; (h) utilizing outside resources from the community, friends, and other kin; and (i) refraining from the use of violence and drugs. Though rather idealistic, the Leonards' case illustrates functional family coping.

Across the street from the Leonard family is the Mosher family. Remarkably similar events have occurred in this family, but with differing results. Mr. Mosher's father has died, and his mother required surgery soon after the funeral. Mrs. Mosher recently returned to work at a higher paying job than her husband. In sharp contrast to the Leonards, the Moshers were unable to see their mounting stressors and resulting predicament and tended to deny even to themselves that the death, illness, and return to work were affecting them. The stress they experienced, which resulted in violent outbursts and excessive drinking and smoking by both parents, was (a) blamed on the oldest child's rebellious attitude toward his parents (individual-centered and blame-oriented). This seemingly normative life transition became a crisis for the Moshers because of ineffective methods of coping and was aggravated by (b) their intolerance of each other's behaviors; (c) lack of clear and direct commitment to and affection for each other (leading to various coalitions within the family); (d) closed channels of communication within the family; (e) the maintenance of rigid family roles; and (f) low family cohesion. Making matters even worse was their (g) reluctance to seek outside help.

TABLE 2
Contrast Between Functional and Dysfunctional Family Coping

Characteristics	For Families which are coping	
	Functionally	Dysfunctionally
Identification of the stressor	Clear, Acceptance	Unclear, Denial
Locus of the problem	Family-centered	Individual-centered
Approach to the problem	Solution-oriented	Blame-oriented
Tolerance of others	High	Low
Commitment to and affection for family members	Clear, Direct	Unclear, Indirect
Communication utilization	Open	Closed
Family cohesion	High	Low
Family roles	Flexible, Shifting	Rigid
Resource utilization	Balanced to High	Low to None
Use of violence	Absent	Present
Use of drugs	Infrequent	Frequent

CONCLUSION

Many stressors affecting the family are relatively predictable and common, yet demand considerable family resources to cope effectively on a daily basis. Stress is a fact of life, a natural and expected aspect of emotional and social development. The extent to which families cope with this normative stress is associated with their happiness and comfort. Thus, for some families mounting stress brings them together in a spirit of teamwork and cooperation, mutual need-meeting and support. For other families the stress they experience leads to mounting conflict and a cycle of destructive reactions which may literally destroy the family.

In general, although sources of stress vary, effective reactions to them do not. The chapters in Volume II will further demonstrate the power and effectiveness of families in overcoming and adapting to a wide variety and intensity of stressors. What can we conclude from all of this? As family members we must remind ourselves and our fellow family members that there are, indeed, right and wrong ways of coping with stress and to heed the lessons and models provided by functional families.

Perhaps more importantly, those of us who are in the enterprise of family assistance—be it policy or program formulators, therapists or counselors, researchers or educators—should be familiar with the stress-family connection as we know it and strive to learn more. Our goal should be to *facilitate* family adaptation rather than supplant it and to help families utilize their own natural support systems and coping strategies. Only selectively should we intervene in their coping efforts, when requested, and most often in an advisory capacity.

References

Ackerman, N.W. *The psychodynamics of family life.* New York: Basic Books, 1958.
Ahrons, C.R. The binuclear family: Two households, one family. *Alternative Lifestyles,* 1979, 2, 499-515.
Ahrons, C.R. Divorce: A crisis of family transition and change. *Family Relations,* October, 1980, 29, 533-540.(a)
Ahrons, C.R. Joint custody arrangements in the post-divorce family. *Journal of Divorce,* 1980, 3, 189-205.(b)
Ahrons, C.R. Redefining the divorced family: A conceptual framework for post-divorce family system reorganization. *Social Work,* 1980, 25, 437-441.(c)
Ahrons, C.R. The continuing coparental relationship between divorced spouses. *American Journal of Orthopsychiatry,* 1981, 5, 415-428.
Ahrons, C.R., & Perlmutter, M.S. The relationship between former spouses: A fundamental subsystem in the remarriage family. In L. Messinger (Ed.) *Therapy with Remarriage Families.* Roakville, MD: Aspen Systems Corp., 1982.
Albrecht, R. The parental responsibilities of grandparents. *Marriage and Family Living,* 1954, 16, 201-204.
Aldous, J. *Family careers: Developmental change in families.* New York: John Wiley & Sons, 1978.
Aldous, J., & Hill, R. Breaking the poverty cycle: Strategic points for intervention. *Social Work,* 1969, 14, 3-12.
Anderson, L.S. When a child begins school. *Children Today,* August 1976, 16-19.
Angell, R.C. *The family encounters the Depression.* New York: Charles Scribner, 1936.
Anthony, E.J., & Koupernik, C. (Eds.), *The child in his family: Children at psychiatric risk (Vol. 3).* New York: John Wiley & Sons, 1974.
Antonovsky, A. *Health, stress and coping.* San Francisco, CA: Jossey-Bass, 1979.
Atchley, R.C. Introduction. In R.C. Atchley & T.O. Byerts (Eds.), *Rural environments and aging.* Washington, DC: The Gerontological Society, 1975.
Bachrach, L. *Human services in rural areas: An analytical review.* Rochville, MD: Project Share, 1981.
Baekland, F., & Lundwall, L. Dropping out of treatment: A critical review. *Psychological Bulletin,* 1975, 82, 738-783.
Bahr, S. Effects on power and division of labor in the family. In L. Hoffman & F.I. Nye (Eds.), *Working women.* San Francisco, CA: Jossey-Bass, 1974.
Bakke, E. *Citizens without work.* New Haven, CT: Yale University Press, 1940.
Bakke, E. *The unemployed worker.* New Haven, CT: Yale University Press, 1942.
Ball, R.A. Sociology and general systems theory. *American Sociologist,* 1978, 13, 65-78.
Bane, M. Marital disruption and the lives of children. *Journal of Social Issues,* 1976, 32, 103-117.
Baranowski, M.D. Adolescents' attempted influence on parental behaviors. *Adolescence,* 1978, 13, 585-604.
Barker, R. *Ecological psychology.* Palo Alto, CA: Stanford University Press, 1968.

Barnett, L.D., & MacDonald, R.H. A study of the membership of the National Organization for Nonparents. *Social Biology*, 1976, *23*, 297-310.

Barrett, N.S., & Driscoll, A. The impact of inflation on families. *The Family Economics Review.* Spring, 1976.

Baumrind, D. Child care practices anteceding three patterns of preschool behavior. *Genetic Psychological Monographs*, 1967, *75*, 43-88.

Beale, C.L. *Rural and small town population change, 1970-1980.* Washington, DC: U.S. Department of Agriculture Economics and Statistics Service, February, 1981.

Bennett, S.K., & Elder, G.H., Jr. Women's work in the family economy: A study of Depression hardship in women's lives. *Journal of Family History*, 1979, *4*, 153-176.

Berman, W.H., & Turk, D.C. Adaptation to divorce: Problems and coping strategies. *Journal of Marriage and the Family*, 1981, *43*, 1-139.

Bernard, J. *Remarriage.* New York: Holt, Rinehart, & Winston, 1956.

Bernard J. The eudaemonists. In S.Z. Klausner (Ed.), *Why man makes changes.* Garden City, NY: Doubleday & Company, 1968.

Bernard, J. *The future of motherhood.* New York: Penguin Books, 1974.

Bernard, J. *Women, wives, mothers.* Chicago: Aldine Publishing Company, 1975.

Bescher-Donnelly, L., & Smith, L.W. The changing roles and status of rural women. In R.T. Coward & W.M. Smith, Jr. (Eds.), *The family in rural society.* Boulder, CO: Westview Press, 1981, 167-185.

Billingsley, A. *Black families in white America.* Englewood Cliffs, NJ: Prentice-Hall, 1968.

Blackwood, L.G., & Carpenter, E.H. The importance of anti-urbanism in determining residential preference and migration patterns. *Rural Sociology*, 1978, *43*, 31-47.

Blood, R.O., & Wolfe, D.M. *Husbands and wives: The dynamics of married living.* Glencoe, IL: The Free Press, 1960.

Bloom, B.L., & Caldwell, R.A. Sex differences in adjustment during the process of marital separation. *Journal of Marriage and the Family*, 1981, *43*, 693-701.

Bohannan, P. (Ed.) *Divorce and after.* New York: Anchor Books, 1971.

Boss, P. *Psychological father absence and presence: A theoretical formulation for an investigation into family systems interaction.* Doctoral dissertation. University of Wisconsin, Madison, August 1975.

Boss, P. A clarification of the concept of psychological father presence in families experiencing ambiguity of boundary. *Journal of Marriage and the Family*, 1977, *39*, 141-151.

Boss, P. Normative family stress: Family boundary changes across the life-span. *Family Relations*, October 1980, 445-450.

Boss, P. The relationship of wife's sex role perceptions, psychological father presence, and functioning in the ambiguous father-absent MIA family. *Journal of Marriage and the Family*, 1980(a), *42*, 541-549.

Boss, P. Normative family stress: Family boundary changes across the life-span. *Family Relations*, 1980(b), *29*, 445-450.

Boss, P., McCubbin, H.I., & Lester, G. The corporate executive wife's coping patterns in response to routine husband-father absence. *Family Process*, March 1979, *18*, 79-86.

Boss, P.G., & Whitaker, C. Dialogue on separation. *The Family Coordinator*, 1979, *28*, 391-398.

Bould, S. Female-headed families: Personal fate control and the provider role. *Journal of Marriage and the Family*, 1977, *39*, 339-349.

Boulding, E. Family adjustment to war separation and reunion. *Annals of the American Academy of Political and Social Science*, 1950, *272*, 59-68.

Brandwein, R., Brown, C., & Fox, E. Women and children last: Social situation of divorced mothers and their families. *Journal of Marriage and the Family*, 1974, *36*, 498-514.

Brassard, J. *Ecology of divorce: Case study analysis of personal and social networks and mother-child interaction in divorced and married families.* Paper presented at National Council on Family Relations Annual Meeting, Boston, 1979.

Brim, O.G., Jr. *Education for childrearing.* New York: Russell Sage Foundation, 1959.

Broderick, C., & Smith, J. The general systems approach to the family. In W.R. Burr, R. Hill, F.I. Nye & I.L. Reiss (Eds.), *Contemporary theories about the family, Vol 2.* New York: The Free Press, 1979.

Bronfenbrenner, U. *The changing American family.* Mimeographed. Ithaca, NY: Cornell University, 1974.

Bronfenbrenner, U. The experimental ecology of education. *Educational Researcher,* 1976, *5,* 5-15.

Bronfenbrenner, U. *The ecology of human development.* Cambridge, MA: Harvard University Press, 1980.

Brooks, A. Job help for wives. *New York Times,* 30 August 1981, *III,* 8.

Brown, E. A model of the divorce process. *Conciliation Courts Review,* 1976, *14,* 1-11.

Brown, P. & Manela, R. Changing family roles: Women and divorce. *Journal of Divorce,* 1978, *1,* 315-328.

Bryson, R., Bryson, J., & Johnson, M. Family size, satisfaction, and productivity in dual-career couples. In J.B. Bryson & R. Bryson (Eds.), *Dual-career couples.* New York: Human Sciences, 1978.

Buehler, C., & Hogan, M. Managerial behavior and stress in families headed by divorced women. *Family Relations,* October 1980, *29,* 535-532.

Bulatto, R.A. *The value of children: A cross-national study (Vol. II, The Philippines).* Honolulu, HA: East-West Population Institute, 1975.

Burgess, A.W. & Baldwin, B.A. *Crisis intervention theory and practice: A clinical handbook.* Englewood Cliffs, NJ: Prentice-Hall, 1981.

Burke, R., & Weir, T. Husband-wife helping relationships as moderators of experienced stress: The 'mental hygiene' function of marriage. In H. McCubbin, E. Cauble, & J. Patterson (Eds.), *Family stress, coping and social support.* Springfield, IL: Charles C. Thomas Publisher, 1982.

Burns, K., & Freedman, S. In support of families under stress: A community based approach. *The Family Coordinator,* 1976, *25,* 41-46.

Burnside, B. Gender roles and lifestyles: A sociocultural study of voluntary childlessness. *Dissertation Abstracts International,* March 1978, *38,* 5557-5558.

Burr, W. *Theory construction and the sociology of the family.* New York: John Wiley & Sons, 1973.

Burr, W. *Successful marriage.* Homewood, IL: The Dorsey Press, 1976.

Campbell, A. Subjective measures of well-being. *American Psychologist,* 1976, *31,* 117-124.

Campbell, A., Converse, P., & Rodgers, W. *The quality of American life.* New York: Russell Sage Foundation, 1976.

Cannon-Bonvente, K., & Kahn, J.R. *The ecology of help-seeking behavior among adolescent parents.* Cambridge, MA: American Institute for Research, 1979.

Caplan, G. *American handbook of psychiatry (Vol. 2).* New York: Basic Books, 1974.

Caplan, G., & Killilea, M. (Eds.), *Support systems and mutual help.* New York: Grune & Stratton, 1976.

Caplovitz, D. *Making ends meet.* Beverly Hills, CA: Sage Publications, 1979.

Carlson, J., Lassey, M., & Lassey, W. *Rural society and environment in America.* New York: McGraw-Hill Book Company, 1981.

Catalyst. *Corporations and two-career families: Directions for the future.* New York, 1981.

Cavan, R., & Ranck, K. *The family and the Depression.* Chicago: University of Chicago Press, 1938.

Chilman, C. Some psychosocial aspects of female sexuality. *The Family Coordinator,* 1974, *23,* 123-132.

Chiriboga, D., Coho, A., Stein, J.A., & Roberts, J. Divorce, stress and social supports: A study in helpseeking behavior. *Journal of Divorce,* 1979, *2,* 121-135.

Church, J. *Understanding your child from birth to three: A guide to your child's psychological development.* New York: Pocket Books, 1976.

Citizens Advisory Council on the Status of Women. *Memorandum: The Equal Rights Amend-*

ment and alimony and child support laws. Washington, DC: U.S. Government Printing Office, January 1972.

Clarke-Stewart, A. Popular primers for parents. *American Psychologist,* 1978, *33,* 359-369.

Cleveland, M. Sex in marriage: At 40 and beyond. *The Family Coordinator,* 1974, *23,* 123-132.

Cobb, S. Social support as a moderator of life stress. *Psychosomatic Medicine,* 1976, *38,* 300-314.

Cofer, C., & Appley, M. *Motivation: Theory and research.* New York: John Wiley & Sons, 1964.

Colletta, N. Support systems after divorce: Incidence and impact. *Journal of Marriage and the Family,* November 1979, *4,* 837-846.

Colletta, N. *The influence of support systems on the maternal behavior of young mothers.* Paper presented at the Society for Research in Child Development Biennial Meeting, Boston, Massachusetts, April, 1981.

Collins, A., & Pancoast, D. *Natural helping networks: A strategy for prevention.* Washington, DC: National Association for Social Workers, 1976.

Couch, S. Women and work: Historical perspective. *Tips and Topics,* Summer 1980, *20.*

Cowan, C., Cowan, P., Coie, L., & Coie, J. Becoming a family: The impact of a first child's birth on the couple's relationship. In W. Miller, L. Newman (Eds.), *The first child and family formation.* Chapel Hill, NC: Carolina Population Center, University of North Carolina, 1978.

Coward, R.T. Rural families changing but retain distinctiveness. *Rural Development Perspectives,* 1980, *3,* 4-8.

Coward, R.T. Demythologizing the farm family. *Catholic Rural Life,* 1981, *31,* 16-20.

Coward, R.T. Family life in small towns and rural communities: Persistence, change and diversity. In R. Craycroft (Ed.), *Change and tradition in the American small town.* Starksboro, MS: University Press of Mississippi, 1982.

Coward, R.T., & Smith, W.M., Jr. (Eds.). *The family in rural socity.* Boulder, CO: Westview Press, 1981.

Coward R.T., & Smith, W.M., Jr. Families in rural society. In D.A. Dillman & D.J. Hobbs (Eds.), *Rural society in the U.S.: Issues for the 1980s.* Boulder, CO: Westview Press, 1982.

Crnic, K.A., Greenberg, M.T., Ragozin, A.S., & Robinson, N.M. *The effects of life stress and social support on the life satisfaction and attitudes of mothers of newborn normal and at-risk infants.* Paper presented at the annual conference of the Western Psychological Association, Honolulu, May 1980.

Crnic, K.A., Greenberg, M.T., Ragozin, A.S., Robinson, N.M., & Basham, R. *The effects of stress and social support on maternal attitudes and the mother-infant relationship.* Paper presented at the Society for Research in Child Development Biennial Meeting, Boston, April 1981.

Cronenwett, L. Elements and outcomes of a postpartum support group. *Research in Nursing and Health,* 1980, *3,* 33-41.

Culbert, S., & Renshaw, J. Coping with the stresses of travel as an opportunity for improving the quality of work and family life. *Family Process,* 1972, *11,* 321-337.

Dalzell, I. Evaluation of a prenatal teaching program. *Nursing Research,* 1965, *14,* 160-163.

Deacon, R., & Firebaugh, F. *Home Management: Context and concepts.* Boston, MA: Houghton, Mifflin, 1975.

Deacon, R., & Firebaugh, F. *Family resource management.* Boston, MA: Allyn & Bacon, 1981.

Deutscher, I. The quality of postparental life. *Journal of Marriage and the Family,* 1964, *26,* 52-59.

Doering, S., & Entwisle, R. Preparation during pregnancy and ability to cope with labor and delivery. *American Journal of Orthopsychiatry,* 1975, *45,* 825-837.

Dohrenwend, B.S., & Dohrenwend, B.P. *Stressful life events.* New York: John Wiley & Sons, 1974.

References   233

Drabeck, T., Key, W., Erickson, P., & Kaplan, B. The impact of disaster on kin relationships. *Journal of Marriage and the Family*, August 1975, 37, 481-494.
Dresen, S.E. The sexually active middle adult. *American Journal of Nursing*, 1975, 75, 1001-1005.
Drotar, D., Baskiewicz, A., Irvin, N., Kennell, J., & Klaus, M. The adaptation of parents to the birth of an infant with a congenital malformation: A hypothetical model. *Pediatrics*, 1967, 40, 596-602.
Duberman, L. *The reconstituted family: A study of remarried couples and their children*. Chicago: Nelson-Hall, 1975.
Dudrow, J., Fowler, R., & Wallace, D. *Northwestern National Bank of Minneapolis work and family research study*. Paper presented at Annual Meeting, National Council on Family Relations, Milwaukee, 1981.
Duncan, G.J. An overview of family economic mobility. *Economic Outlook USA*, 1981, 8, 65-67.
Duncan, G.J. Unmarried heads of households and marriage. In G.F. Duncan and J. Morgan (Eds.), *Five thousand American families: Patterns of economic progress*. Ann Arbor, MI: Institute for Social Research, 1975.
Duvall E. *Family development*. Philadelphia, PA: Lippincott & Co., 1977.
Dyer, E.D. Parenthood as crisis: A restudy. *Marriage and Family Living*, 1963, 25, 196-201.
Eaton, W. Life events, social supports and psychiatric symptoms: A re-analysis of the New Haven data. *Journal of Health and Social Behavior*, 1978, 19, 230-234.
Elder, G.H., Jr. *Children of the Great Depression*. Chicago: University of Chicago Press, 1974.
Elder, G.H., Jr. Scarcity and prosperity in postwar childbearing: Explorations from a life course perspective. *Journal of Family History*, 1981, 6, 410-433.
Entwisle, R., & Doering, S. *The first birth*. Baltimore, MD: The Johns Hopkins University Press, 1980.
Epstein, C. Law partners and marital partners: Strains and solutions in the dual-career family enterprise. *Human Relations*, 1971, 24, 549-563.
Erikson, E.H. *Childhood and society*. New York: W.W. Norton & Company, 1950.
Erikson, E.H. Identity and the life cycle. *Psychological Issues*, 1959, 1, 18-164.
Erikson, E.H. Youth: fidelity and diversity, In E.H. Erikson, (Ed.), *Youth: Change and challenge*. New York: Basic Books, 1963.
Erikson, E.H. *Identity, youth and crisis*. New York: W.W. Norton & Company, 1968.
Erikson, E.H. (Ed.) *Adulthood*. New York: W.W. Norton, 1976.
Erikson, K. *Everything in its path: Destruction of the community in the Buffalo Creek flood*. New York: Simon & Schuster, 1976.
Espenshade, T. The economic consequences of divorce. *Journal of Marriage and the Family*,1979, 41, 615-625.
Espenshade, T. Raising a child can now cost $85,000. *Intercom (Population Reference Bureau)*, September 1980, 8, 10-13.
Farber, B. *Family organization and interaction*. San Francisco: Chandler Publishing Company, 1964.
Farmer, L. *Remarks made at the Second Chatauqua in Mississippi, "Change and tradition in the American small town."* Mississippi: State University, April 1981.
Fast, I., & Cain, A. The stepparent role: Potential for disturbances in family functioning. *American Journal of Orthopsychiatry*, April 1966, 36, 485-491.
Fawcett, J. *The satisfactions and costs of children: Theories, concepts, methods*. Honolulu, HA: East-West Population Center, 1972.
Feinberg, M. *Corporate bigamy*. New York: William Morrow & Company, 1980.
Feldman, H. *Development of the husband-wife relationship*. Unpublished manuscript, Cornell University, 1965.
Feldman, H. The effects of children on the family. In A. Michel (Ed.), *Family issues of employed women in Europe and America*. W.Leiden, Netherlands: E.J. Brill, 1971.

Figley, C.R. Child density and the marital relationship. *Journal of Marriage and the Family*, 1973, *35*(2), 272-282.

Figley, C.R. The Iran crisis: Caring for families of catastrophe. *Family Therapy News*, 1980(September 4-5), 5-6.

Figley, C.R. Family absorption of catastrophic stress: Case of the Iran Hostage families. Invited address, St. Joseph College(Indiana), March, 1981.

Figley, C.R. Traumatization and comfort: Close relationships may be hazardous to your health. Invited address, Texas Tech University(Lubbock, Texas), February, 1982.

Fitchen, J. *Poverty in rural America: A case study.* Boulder, CO: Westview Press, 1981.

Flavell, J.H. *The developmental psychology of Jean Piaget.* New York: Van Nostand, 1963.

Flavell, J.H. Metacognition and cognitive monitoring: A new area of cognitive-developmental inquiry. *American Psychologist*, 1979, *34*, 906-911.

Folberg, J., & Graham, M. *Joint custody of children following divorce.* Law Review, University of California, Davis, 1979.

Ford, T.R. (Ed.) *Rural USA: Persistence and change.* Ames, IA: Iowa State University Press, 1978.

Fried, S., & Holt, P. Parent education: One strategy for the prevention of child abuse. In M.J. Fine (Ed.), *Handbook on parent education.* New York: Academic Press, 1980.

Friedan, B. *The second stage.* New York: Summit Books, 1981.

Fullerton, H. The 1995 labor force: A first look. *Monthly Labor Review*, December 1980, 11-21.

Furstenberg, F. Jr. Recycling the family: Perspectives for a neglected family form. *Marriage & Family Review*, 1979, *2*, 12-22.

Gagnon, J. Sexuality and sexual learning in the child. *Psychiatry*, 1965, *28*, 212-228.

Gasser, R., & Taylor, C. Role adjustment of single-parent fathers with dependent children. *The Family Coordinator*, 1976, *25*, 397-401.

Geboy, M. Who is listening to the "experts?" The use of child care materials by parents. *Family Relations*, 1981, *30*, 205-210.

George, L. *Role transitions in later life.* Belmont, CA: Brooks/Cole, 1980.

General Mills American Family Report. *Raising children in a changing society.* Minneapolis, MN: General Mills, 1977.

General Mills American Family Report. *Family health in an era of stress.* Minneapolis, MN: General Mills, 1979.

General Mills American Family Report. *Families at work: Strengths & Strains.* Minneapolis, MN: General Mills, 1981.

Geretal, N., & Gross, H. *A special case of dual-career families and couples who live apart.* Paper presented at Groves Conference on Marriage and Family, Mt. Pocono, PA, 1981.

Gilbert, L., Holahan, C., & Manning, L. Coping with conflict between professional and maternal roles. *Family Relations*, 1981, *30*, 419-426.

Glasser, P., & Navarre, E. Structural problems of the one-parent family. *Journal of Social Issues*, 1965, *211*, 98-109.

Glenn, N. Psychological well-being in the postparental stage: Some evidence from national surveys. *Journal of Marriage and the Family*, 1975, *37*, 105-110.

Glick, P. The life cycle of the family. *Marriage and Family Living*, 1955, *17*, 3-9.

Glick, P. A demographic picture of black families. In H. McAdoo (Ed.), *Black families.* Beverly Hills, CA: Sage Publications, 1981.

Golan, N. *Passing through transitions.* New York: The Free Press, 1981.

Goldstein, J., Freud, A., & Solnit A. *Beyond the best interests of the child.* New York: The Free Press, 1973.

Goode, W. *After divorce.* New York: The Free Press, 1956.

Goodman, E. The new ideal American woman. In L. Van Gelder, *Ellen Goodman: A columnist you can trust.* Ms, March 1979.

Goodman, E. To work or not: Women's dilemma. *Minneapolis Tribune*, 7 April, 1981, *10*.

Gore, S. The effect of social support in moderating the health consequences of unemployment. *Journal of Health and Social Behavior*, June 1978, *19*, 157-165.

Gottesman, R. (Ed.) Our children and the law. *Children's Legal Rights Journal*. Washington, DC: Children's Legal Rights Information and Training Program, 1981.

Gottleib, B.H., & Schroter C. Collaboration and resources exchange between professionals and natural support systems. *Professional Psychologist*, November 1978, 614-622.

Granovetter, M. The strength of weak ties. *American Journal of Sociology*, 1973, *78*, 1360-1380.

Greiff, B., & Munter, P. *Tradeoffs*. New York: New American Library, 1980.

Grief, J. Father, children and joint custody. *American Journal of Orthopsychiatry*, 1979, *49*, 311-319.

Grossman, A. Working mothers and their children. *Monthly Labor Review*, May 1981, 49-54.

Grote, D. & Weinstein, J. Joint custody: A viable and ideal alternative. *Journal of Divorce*, 1977, *1*, 43-53.

Guadagno, M.A.N. *A systems approach to family financial management: Implications for family research*. Paper presented at the Theory Development and Methods Workshop, National Council on Family Relations, Milwaukee, 1981.

Gullotta, T., & Donohue, K. The corporate family: Theory and treatment. *The Journal of Marital and Family Therapy*, April 1981, *7*, 151-158.

Haan, N. *Coping and defending: Processes of self-environment organization*. New York: Academic Press, 1977.

Hadley, T.R., Jacob, T., Millones, J., Caplan, J., & Spitz, D. The relationship between family development crisis and the appearance of symptoms in a family member. *Family Process*, 1974, 207-214.

Haley, J. *Leaving home: The therapy of disturbed young people*. New York: McGraw-Hill, 1980.

Hampton, R. Marital disruption: Some social and economic consequences. In G.J. Duncan and J.N. Morgan, (Eds.), *Five thousand American families: Patterns of economic progress (Vol. 3)*. Ann Arbor, MI: Institute for Social Research, 1975.

Hansen, D., & Hill, R. Families under stress. In H.T. Christensen (Ed.), *Handbook of marriage and the family*. Chicago: Rand McNally & Company, 1964.

Hansen, D., & Johnson, V. Rethinking family stress theory: Definitional aspects. In W. Burr, R. Hill, I. Nye, & I. Reiss (Eds.), *Contemporary theories about the family (Vol. 1)*. New York: The Free Press, 1979.

Harman, D., & Brim, O., Jr. *Learning to be parents: Principles, programs, and methods*. Beverly Hills, CA: Sage Publications, 1980.

Havighurst, R. *Human development and education*. London, England: Longmans, Green, 1953.

Havighurst, R. *Developmental tasks and education*. New York: McKay, 1972.

Hayghe, H. Working wives' contribution to family income in 1977. *Monthly Labor Review*, October 1979.

Hayghe, H. Husbands and wives as earners: An analysis of family data. *Monthly Labor Review*, February 1981.

Heckman, N., Bryson, R., & Bryson, J. Problems of professional couples: A content analysis. *Journal of Marriage and the Family*, 1977, *39*, 323-330.

Helfer, R., & Kempe, C. (Eds.) *Child abuse and neglect: The family and the community*. Cambridge, MA: Ballinger, 1976.

Herzog, E., & Sudia, C. Children in fatherless families. In B. Caldwell & H. Ricciuti (Eds.), *Review of child development research*. Chicago: University of Chicago Press, 1973.

Hess, G., & Handel, G. *Family worlds: The psychosocial interior of the family*. Chicago: University of Chicago Press, 1974.

Hetherington, E.M. Divorce: A child's perspective. *American Psychologist*, October 1979, *34*, 851-858.

Hetherington, E.M., Cox, M., & Cox, R. Divorced fathers. *The Family Coordinator,* 1976, 25, 417-428.

Hetherington, E.M., & Deur, J. The effects of father absence on child development. *Young Children,* 1971, 26, 233-248.

Hill, R. *Families under stress.* New York: Harper & Row, 1949.

Hill, R. Generic features of families under stress. *Social Casework,* 1958, 49, 139-150.

Hill, R. Challenges and resources for family development. In *Family mobility in our dynamic society.* Ames, IA: Iowa State University, 1965.

Hill, R. *Family development in three generations: A longitudinal study of changing family patterns of planning and achievement.* Cambridge, MA: Schenkman, 1970.

Hill, R., & Joy, C. *Conceptualizing and operationalizing category systems for phasing family development.* Unpublished paper. 1979.

Hill, Robert. *The strengths of the Black Family.* Washington, DC: National Urban League, 1971.

Hirshey, G. "Ma, there's a computer in the kitchen!" *Family Circle,* September 22, 1981.

Hite, S. *The Hite report: A nationwide study of female sexuality.* New York: Macmillan Publishing Company, 1976.

Hobbs, D., Jr. Parenthood as crisis: A third study. *Journal of Marriage and the Family,* 1965, 27, 367-372.

Hobbs, D., Jr. Transition to parenthood: A replication and an extension. *Journal of Marriage and the Family.* 1968, 30, 413-417.

Hobbs, D., Jr., & Cole, S. Transition to parenthood: A decade replication. *Journal of Marriage and the Family,* 1976, 38, 723-731.

Hobbs, D., Jr., & Wimbish, J. Transition to parenthood by Black couples. *Journal of Marriage and the Family,* 1977, 39, 677-689.

Hoffman, L. Effects on child. In L. Hoffman & I. Nye (Eds.), *Working mothers.* San Francisco, CA: Jossey-Bass, 1974.

Hoffman, L., & Manis, J. The value of children in the United States: A new approach to the study of fertility. *Journal of Marriage and the Family,* 1979, 41, 583-596.

Hollister, R., & Palmer, J. The impact of inflation on the poor. In K. Boulding & M. Pfaff (Eds.), *Redistribution of the rich and poor: The grants economics of income redistribution (Vol. 1).* Belmont, CA: Wadsworth Publishing Company, 1972.

Holmes, T., & Rahe, R. The Social Readjustment Rating Scale. *Journal of Psychosomatic Research,* 1967, 11, 213-218.

Holmstrom, L. *The two-career family.* Cambridge, MA: Schenkman, 1973.

Honeywell Women's Task Force. *Child care recommendations for Honeywell employees.* July 1980.

Honeywell Working Parents' Task Force. *Preliminary report and recommendations.* August 1981.

Hooper, J.O. My wife, the student. *The Family Coordinator,* 1979, 28, 459-464.

Hungerford, M. *Childbirth education.* Springfield, IL: Charles C. Thomas Publishers, 1972.

Hyman, H., & Reed J. Black matriarchy reconsidered: Evidence from secondary analysis of sample surveys. *Public Opinion Quarterly,* 1969, 33, 346-354.

Inhelder, B., & Piaget, J. *The growth of logical thinking from childhood to adolescence.* New York: Basic Books, 1958.

Institute for the Study of Educational Policy. *Minorities in two-year colleges.* Washington, D.C.: Howard University, 1980.

Jacoby, A. Transition to parenthood: A reassessment. *Journal of Marriage and the Family,* 1969, 31, 720-727.

Janis, I.L. Stress and Frustration. *Personality variables in social behavior.* New York: Harcourt Brace Jovanovich, 1971.

Janis, I.L., & Leventhal, H. Human reactions to stress. In E. Borgatta & W. Lambert (Eds.), *Handbook of personality theory and research.* Chicago: Rand McNally, 1968.

Janis, L., & Mann, L. *Decision making: A psychological analysis of conflict, choice, and com-*

mitment. New York: The Free Press, 1977.

Jauch, C. The one-parent family. *Journal of Clinical Child Psychology,* 1977, 30-32.

Johnson, B. Changes in marital and family characteristics of workers, 1970-1978. *Monthly Labor Review,* April 1979.

Johnson, B. Marital and family characteristics of the labor force, March 1979. *Monthly Labor Review,* April 1980,

Jones, L. *Great expectations: America and the baby boom generation.* New York: Coward, McCann & Geohagan, 1971.

Juster, F. Why do consumers fear inflation? *ISR Newsletter,* Spring 1979.

Kaplan, H. *The new sex therapy: Active treatment of sexual dysfunctions.* New York: Brunner/Mazel, 1974.

Kaplan. H., *Disorders of sexual desire: The new sex therapy (Vol. 2).* New York: Brunner/Mazel, 1979.

Katz, A. Self-help organizations and volunteer participation in social welfare. *Social Work,* 1970, *15,* 15-20.

Kaufman, J. Black managers. *Wall Street Journal,* 9 July 1980, 1.

Kempe, C., & Helfer, R. (Eds.), *Helping the battered child and his family.* Philadelphia: Lippincott & Company, 1974.

Keshet, H. & Rosenthal, K. Fathering after marital separation. *Social Work,* 1978, *23,* 11-18.

Kiell, N. *The universal experience of adolescence.* New York: International Universities Press, Inc., 1964.

Kitson, G., & Raschke, H. A review of research on divorce: What we know, what we need to know. *Journal of Divorce,* 1981.

Kitson, G., & Sussman, M. *The processes of marital separation and divorce: Male and female similarities and differences.* Paper presented at the meetings of the American Sociological Association, New York, August 1976.

Klein, D.C., & Ross, A. Kindergarten entry: A study of role transition. In M. Krugman (Ed.), *Orthopsychiatry and the school.* New York: American Orthopsychiatric Association, 1958.

Komarovsky, M. *The unemployed man and his family.* New York: Dryden Press, 1940.

Komopka, G. Requirements for healthy development of adolescent youth. *Adolescence,* 1973, *8,* 291-316.

Koos, E. *Families in trouble.* New York: King's Crown Press, 1946.

Kressel, K., & Deutsch, M. Divorce therapy: An in-depth survey of therapists' views. *Family Process,* 1977, *16,* 413-443.

Lamb, M. The effects of divorce on children's personality development. *Journal of Divorce,* 1977, *1,* 163-174.

Larossa, R., & Larossa, M. *Transition to parenthood: How infants change families.* Beverly Hills, CA: Sage Publications, 1981.

Lawe, C., & Lawe, B. The balancing act: Coping strategies for emerging family lifestyles. In F. Pepitone-Rockwell (Ed.), *Dual-career families.* Beverly Hills, CA: Sage Publications, 1980.

Lazarus, R. *Psychological stress and the coping process.* New York: McGraw-Hill Book Company, 1966.

Lazarus, R. Positive denial: The case of not facing reality. *Psychology Today,* November, 1979.

Lee, G. Effects of social networks on the family. In W. Burr, R. Hill, F.I. Nye & I. Reiss (Eds.), *Contemporary theories about the family (Vol. 1).* New York: The Free Press, 1979.

Lee, G., & Cassidy, M.L. Kinship systems and extended family ties. In R.T. Coward & W.M. Smith, Jr (Eds.), *The family in rural society.* Boulder, CO: Westview Press, 1981.

LeMasters, E. Parenthood as crisis. *Marriage and Family Living,* 1957, *19,* 352-355.

LeMasters, E. *Parents in modern America.* Homewood, IL: The Dorsey Press, 1970.

Levine, J. *Who will raise the children?* Philadelphia, PA: J.B. Lippincott, 1976.

Levinson, D. with Darrow, C.N., Klein, E.B., Levinson, M.H., & McKee, B. *The seasons of a man's life.* New York: Alfred A. Knopf, 1978.

Levitan, S., & Belous, R. Work-sharing initiatives at home and abroad. *Monthly Labor Review,* September 1977.

Lewis, R., Freneau, P., & Roberts, C. Fathers and the post-parental transition. *The Family Coordinator,* 1979, *41,* 514-520.

Lewis, J.M., Beavers, W.R., Gossett, J.T., & Phillips, V.A. *No single thread: Psychological health in family systems.* New York: Brunner/Mazel, 1976.

Lieberman, M., Berman, L., & Associates. *Self-help groups for coping in crisis.* San Francisco: Jossey-Bass, 1979.

Lifton, R.J. *The broken connection.* New York: Simon & Schuster, 1979.

Lin, N., Simeone, R., Ensel, W., & Kuo, W. Social support, stressful life events and illness: A model and an empirical test. *Journal of Health and Social Behavior,* 1979, *20,* 108-119.

Lipman-Blumen, J. A crisis framework applied to macrosociological family changes: Marriage, divorce, and occupational trends associated with World War II. *Journal of Marriage and the Family,* 1975, *3,* 889-902.

Litwak, E. & Szelenyi, I. Primary group structures and their functions: Kin, neighbors and friends. *American Sociological Review,* 1969, *34,* 465-481,

Longfellow, C., Zelkowitz, P., Saunders, E., & Belle, D. *The role of support in moderating the effects of stress and depression.* Paper presented at the Society for Research in Child Development Biennial Meeting, San Francisco, March 1979.

Lopata, H. *Widowhood in an American city.* Cambridge, MA: Schenkman, 1973.

Lopata, H. Contributions of extended families to the support systems of metropolitan area widows: Limitations of modified kin networks. *Journal of Marriage and the Family,* 1978, *40,* 355-366.

Lopata, H. *Women as widows.* New York: Elsevier, 1979.

LoPiccolo, J., & LoPiccolo, L. (Eds.), *Handbook of sex therapy.* New York: Plenum Press, 1978.

Luepnitz, D. Children of divorce: A review of the psychological exercise. *Law and Human Behavior,* 1978, *2,* 167-179.

Machlowitz, M. *Workaholics.* Boston, MA: Addison-Wesley Publishing, 1980.

Mack, D. Where the Black matriarchy theorists went wrong. *Psychology Today,* January 1971.

Magrab, P. For the sake of the children: A review of the psychological effects of divorce. *Journal of Divorce,* 1978, *1,* 233-245.

Maguire, L. The interface of social workers with personal networks. *Social Work with Groups,* 1980, *3,* 39-49.

Marcia, J.E. Development and validation of ego-identity status. *Journal of Personality and Social Psychology,* 1966, *3,* 551-558.

Masters, W.H., & Johnson, V.E. *Human sexual response.* Boston: Little, Brown, 1966.

Masters, W.H., & Johnson, V.E. *Human sexual inadequacy.* Boston: Little, Brown, 1970.

Maynard, P., Maynard, N., McCubbin, H., & Shao, D. Family life and the police profession: Coping patterns wives employ in managing job stress and the family environment. *Family Relations,* October 1980, *29,* 495-502.

McAdoo, H. Factors related to stability in upwardly mobile black families. *Journal of Marriage and the Family,* November 1978, *40,* 762-778.

McAdoo, H. Black kinship. *Psychology Today,* May 1979, 67-69.

McAdoo, Harriette. Demographic trends for people of color. *Social Work,* 1982, *27:1,* 15-23. (a)

McAdoo, H. Levels of stress and family support in black families. In H. McCubbin, E. Cauble, & J. Patterson (Eds.), *Family stress, coping and social support.* Springfield, IL: Charles C. Thomas, 1982. (b)

McArthur, A. Developmental tasks and parent-adolescent conflict. *Marriage and Family Living,* 1962, *24* (May): 189-191.

McCubbin, H.I. Integrating coping behavior in family stress theory. *Journal of Marriage and the Family*, May 1979, *41* 237-244.

McCubbin, H.I., Boss, P., Wilson, L.R., & Lester, G.R. Developing family invulnerability to stress: Coping patterns and strategies wives employ in managing family separations. In J. Trost (Ed.), *The family in change*. Vasters, Sweden: International Library, 1980.

McCubbin, H.I., Dahl, B., & Hunter, E. Research in the military family: A review. In H.I. McCubbin, B. Dahl, & E. Hunter (Eds.), *Families in the military system*. Beverly Hills: Sage Publications, 1976.

McCubbin, H.I., Joy, C.B., Cauble, A.E., Comeau, J.K., Patterson, J.M., & Needle, R.H. Family stress and coping: A decade review. *Journal of Marriage and the Family*, 1980, *42*, 855-872.

McCubbin, H.I., & Patterson, J.M. *Systematic Assessment of family stress, resources and coping: Tools for research, education and clinical intervention*. St. Paul, MN: Family Social Science, 1981.

McCubbin, H.I., & Patterson, J.M. Family adaptation to crisis. In H. McCubbin, E. Cauble, & J. Patterson (Eds.), *Family stress, coping, and social support*. Springfield, IL: Charles C. Thomas Publisher, 1982.

McCubbin, H.I., & Patterson, J.M. The family stress process: A double ABCX model of adjustment and adaptation. In H. McCubbin, M. Sussman, & J. Patterson (Eds.), *Advances and developments in family stress theory and research*. New York: Haworth Press, 1983.

McCubbin, H.I., Patterson, J.M., Bauman, E., & Harris, L.H. *Adolescent-family inventory of life events and changes (A-FILE)*. St. Paul, MN: Family Social Science, 1981.

McCubbin, H.I., Patterson, J.M., & Wilson, L. *Family inventory of life events and changes (FILE) Form C*. St. Paul, MN: Family Social Science, 1981.

McGuire, J.S., & Gottleib, B.H. Social support groups among new parents: An experimental study in primary prevention. *Journal of Clinical Child Psychology*, 1979, 111-115.

McLanahan, S.S., Wedemeyer, N.V., & Adelberg, T. Network structure, social support and psychological well-being in the single-parent family. *Journal of Marriage and the Family*, 1981, *43*, 601-612.

Mechanic, D. Social structure and personal adaptation: Some neglected dimensions. In G.V. Coehlo, D.A. Hamburg, & J.E. Adams (Eds.), *Coping and adaptation*. New York: Basic Books, 1974, 32-44.

Melson, G.F. *Family and environment: An ecosystems perspective*. Minneapolis, MN: Burgess Publishing Company, 1980.

Menaghan, E. Assessing the impact of family transitions on marital experience. In H. McCubbin, E. Cauble, & J. Patterson (Eds.), *Family stress, coping, and social support*. Springfield, IL: Charles C. Thomas, 1982.

Mendes, H. Single fatherhood. *Social Work*, 1976, *21*, 308-312.

Messinger, L. Remarriage between divorced people with children from previous marriages. *Journal of Marriage and Family Counseling*, 1976, *2*, 193-200.

Messinger, L., Walker, K., & Freeman, S. Preparation for remarriage following divorce: The use of group techniques. *American Journal of Orthopsychiatry*, 1978, *48*, 263-272.

Mikhail, A. Stress: A psychophysiological conception. *Journal of Human stress*, 1981, *7*, 9-15.

Miller, B.C. A multivariate developmental model of marital satisfaction. *Journal of Marriage and the Family*, 1976, *38*, 643-657.

Miller, B.C., & Sollie, D.L. Normal stresses during the transition to parenthood. *Family Relations*, 1980, *29*, 29-35.

Miller, J.G. *Living systems*. New York: McGraw-Hill Book Company, 1978.

Miller, W.B., & Newman, L.F. (Eds.), *The first child and family formation*. Chapel Hill, NC: Carolina Population Center, 1978.

Minarik, J.J. Who wins, who loses, from inflation? *The Brookings Bulletin*, Summer 1978, 6-10.

Minuchin, S. *Families and family therapy*. Cambridge, MA: Harvard University Press, 1974.

Modell, J., Furstenberg F., & Hershberg, T. Social change and transitions to adulthood in historical perspective. *Journal of Family History*, 1976, *1*, 7-32.

Moen, P. *Patterns of family stress across the life cycle: Work and income related strains—a case in point.* Paper presented at National Council on Family Relations Annual Meeting, Boston, 1979.

Moen, P., Kain, E., & Elder, G.H., Jr. *Economic conditions and family life: Contemporary and historical perspectives.* Paper prepared for the National Academy of Sciences, Assembly of Behavioral and Social Sciences, Committee on Child Development Research and Public Policy, December 1981.

Moore, D. The body image in pregnancy. *Journal of Nurse-Midwifery*, 1978, *22*, 17-27.

Moore, G., & Hedges, J. Trends in labor and leisure. *Monthly Labor Review*, February 1971.

Morgenbessor, M., & Nehls, N. *Joint custody: An alternative for divorcing families.* Chicago: Nelson Hall, 1981.

Mowatt, M. Group psychotherapy for stepfathers and their wives. *Psychotherapy: Theory, research and practice*, 1972, *9*, 328-331.

Mueller, E. Economic motives for family limitation: A study conducted in Taiwan. *Population Studies*, 1972, *27*, 383-403.

Myers-Walls, J. *Transition to parenthood: The role of anticipatory socialization.* Unpublished Master's Thesis, Purdue University, December 1977.

Myers-Walls, J. *A role theory approach to the transition into parenthood.* Unpublished doctoral dissertation, Purdue University, August 1979.

Myers-Walls, J., & Coward, R.T. Natural helping networks: An alternative for rural family service delivery. In R.T. Coward & W.M. Smith (Eds.), *Rural family services: Status and needs.* Lincoln, NE: University of Nebraska Press, in press.

Nag, M. Economic values of children in an agricultural setting. In J. Fawcett (Ed.), *The satisfactions and costs of children: Theories, concepts, methods.* Honolulu, HA: East-West Population Institute, 1972.

Nass, G., Libby, R., & Fisher, M. *Sexual choices: An introduction to human sexuality.* Monterey, CA: Wadsworth Health Sciences Division, 1981.

National Rural Center, *Rural poverty.* Washington DC: National Rural Center, March 1981.

Nemy, E. *More companies aid employees on adoptions.* New York Times, 18 August 1982, *19*.

Neugarten, B.L. (Ed.) *Middle age and aging.* Chicago: University of Chicago Press, 1968.

Neugarten, B., & Hagestad, G. Age and the life course. In R.H. Binstock & E. Shanas (Eds.) *Handbook on aging and the social sciences.* New York: Van Nostrand Reinhold, 1977.

Newman, B.M., & Newman, P.R. *Development through life: A psychosocial approach.* Homewood, IL: The Dorsey Press, 1979.

Nobles, W. African root and American fruit: The Black Family. *Journal of Social and Behavioral Sciences*, 1974, *20*, 66-77.

Nolan, J., The impact of divorce on children. *Conciliation Courts Review*, 1977, *15*, 25-29.

Norton, A., & Glick, P. Marital instability, past, present and future. *Journal of Social Issues*, 1976, *32*, 5-20.

Nuckolls, K., Kassel, J., & Kaplan, B. Psychosocial assets, life crises and the prognosis of pregnancy. *American Journal of Epidemiology*, 1972, *95*, 431-444.

Oakley, A. *The sociology of housework.* London: Martin Robertson, 1974. (a)

Oakley, A. *Woman's work.* New York: Pantheon, 1974.(b)

Ogbu, J. *Minority education and caste.* New York: Academic Press, 1978.

Olson, D.H., & McCubbin, H.I. The circumplex model of marital and family systems VI: Application to family stress and crisis intervention. In H. I. McCubbin, A.E. Cauble, & J.M. Patterson (Eds.), *Family stress, coping, and social support.* Springfield, IL: Charles C. Thomas, 1982.

Olson, D.H., Russell, C.S., & Sprenkle, D.H. Circumplex Model of marital and family systems II: Empirical studies and clinical intervention. In J. Vincent (Ed.), *Advances in family intervention, assessment and theory.* Greenwich, CT: JAI Press, 1979.

Olson, D.H., Sprenkle, D.H., & Russell, C.S. Circumplex model of marital and family systems I: Cohesion and adaptability dimensions, family types and clinical applications. *Family Process*, 1979, *18*, 3-28.

One Child, Two Homes. *Time*, Jan. 29, 1979, *113*, 61.

Orden S., & Bradburn, N. Working wives and marital happiness. *American Journal of Sociology*, January 1969, 392-407.

Orthner, D.K., Brown, T., & Ferguson, D. Single-parent fatherhood: Emerging lifestyle. *The Family Coordinator*, 1976, *25*, 429-437.

Oser, M. *Texas family journal*. Houston: Texas Institute for Families. 1980.

Paloma, M.M. Role conflicts and the married professional woman. In C. Safilios-Rothschild (Ed.), *Toward a sociology of women*. Lexington, MA: Xerox College Publishing, 1972.

Paolucci, B., Hall, O., & Axinn, N. *Family decision making: An ecosystem approach*. New York: John Wiley & Sons, 1977.

Papanek, H. Men, women and work: Reflections on the two-person career. *American Journal of Sociology*, 1973, *78*, 852-872.

Parad, H.J. (Ed.) *Crisis intervention: Selected readings*. New York: Family Service Association of America, 1965.

Parkes, C. *Bereavement: Studies of Grief in Adult Life*. New York: International Universities Press, 1972.

Pearce, D., & McAdoo, H. *Women and children: Alone and in poverty*. Washington, DC: National Advisory Council on Economic Opportunity, September 1981.

Pearlin, L.I., & Johnson, J.S. Marital status, life strains, depression. *American Sociological Review*, 1977, *42*, 704-715.

Pearlin, L.I., & Schooler, C. The structure of coping. *Journal of Health and Social Behavior*, 1978, *19*, 2-21.

Peters, M. *Nine Black families: A study of household management and childrearing in Black families with working mothers*. Unpublished doctoral dissertation. Harvard University, 1976.

Peters, M. "Making it" Black family style: Building on the strength of Black families. In N. Stinnett, J. DeFrain, K. King, P. Knaub, & G. Rowe (Eds.), *Family strengths 3: Roots of well-being*. Lincoln, NE: University of Nebraska Press, 1981.

Pierce, C. The mundane extreme environment and its effect on learning. In S.C. Brainerd (Ed.), *Learning disabilities: Issues and recommendations for research*. Washington, DC: National Institute of Education, 1975.

Piotrowski, C., *Work and the family system*. New York: Macmillan & Company, 1979.

Pleck, J. The work-family role system. *Social Problems*, 1977, *24*, 417-428.

Pleck, J., Staines, G., & Lang, L. Conflicts between work and family life. *Monthly Labor Review*, March 1980.

Portner, J. *Impact of work on the family*. Minneapolis, MN: Minnesota Council on Family Relations, 1978.

Pratt, L. *Family structure and effective health behavior: The energized family*. Boston MA: Houghton Mifflin Company, 1976.

Pridham, K.F., Hansen, M., & Conrad, H.H. Anticipatory care as problem solving in family medicine and nursing. *Journal of Family Practice*, 1977, *4*, 1077-1081.

Rapoport, R. Normal crisis, family structure, and mental health. *Family Process*, 1963, *2*, 68-80.

Rapoport, R., & Rapoport, R.N. Men, women, and equity. *The Family Coordinator*, 1975, *24*, 421-432.

Rapoport, R., & Rapoport, R.N. Dual-career families re-examined. New York: Harper & Row, 1976.

Rapoport, R.N., & Rapoport, R. Dual-career families: Progress and prospects. *Marriage and Family Review*, 1978, *1*, 1-12.

Rapoport, R., & Rapoport, R. Three generations of dual-career family research. In F. Pepitone-Rockwell (Ed.), *Dual-career couples*. Beverly Hills, CA: Sage Publications, 1980.

Rapoport, R., Rapoport, R.N., & Strelitz, Z. *Fathers, mothers and society.* New York: Basic Books, 1977.

Raschke, H.J. *Social and psychological factors in voluntary post-marital dissolution adjustment.* Unpublished doctoral dissertation. University of Minnesota, 1974.

Raschke, H.J. Role of social particpation on post-separation and post-divorce adjustment. *Journal of Divorce,* 1977, *1,* 129-139.

Raschke, H.J. *The development of a post separation/post-divorce problems and stress scale.* Prepared for the National Council on Family Relations Annual Meeting, held in Philadelphia, PA, October 1978.

Reiss, D., & Oliveri, M.E. Family paradigm and family coping: A proposal for linking the family's intrinsic adaptive capacities to its responses to stress. *Family Relations,* 1980, *29,* 431-444.

Reiss, P.J. The extended kinship system: Correlates of and attitudes in frequency of interaction. *Marriage and Family Living,* 1962, *24,* 333-339.

Renee, K.S. Correlates of dissatisfaction in marriage. *Journal of Marriage and the Family,* 1970, *32,* 54-66.

Rice, D. *Dual-career marriage: Conflict and treatment.* New York: The Free Press, 1979.

Rice, F.P. *Dual-career marriage: Marriage and parenthood.* Boston, MA: Allyn & Bacon, 1979.

Richardson, B. *Racism and child rearing.* Unpublished doctoral dissertation, Claremont College, 1981.

Ridley, C.A. Exploring the impact of work satisfaction and involvement on marital interaction when both partners are employed. *Journal of Marriage and the Family,* 1973, *35,* 229-237.

Riegel, K.F. Adult life crises: A dialectical interpretation of development. In N. Datan & L.H. Ginsberg (Eds.), *Life span developmental psychology: Normative life crises.* New York: Academic Press, 1975.

Riegel, K.F. The dialectics of human development. *American Psychologist,* 1976, *31,* 689-699.

Robbins, L., Britton, S., Coats, A.W., Friedman, M., Jay., P., & Laidler, D. *Inflation: Causes, consequences and cures.* London: The Institute of Economic Affairs, 1974.

Robinson, B. Where are you now, Solomon, now that we need you? Criteria in determining child custody. In *Child custody: Literature review and alternative approaches.* Minneapolis, MN: Child Custody Research Project, Hennepin County Domestic Relations Division, 1979.

Rodgers, R. *Family interaction and transaction: The developmental approach.* Englewood Cliffs, NJ: Prentice-Hall, 1973.

Rollins, B.C., & Cannon, K.L. Marital satisfaction over the life cycle: A re-evaluation. *Journal of Marriage and the Family,* 1974, *36,* 271-282.

Rollins, B.C., & Feldman, H. Marital satisfaction over the family life cycle. *Journal of Marriage and the Family,* 1970, *32,* 20-27.

Roman, M., & Haddad, W. *The disposable parent.* New York: Holt, Rinehart & Winston, 1978.

Roosevelt, R., & Lofas, J. *Living in step: A remarriage manual for parents and children.* New York: McGraw-Hill Book Company, 1976.

Rosenblatt, P. Behavior in public places: Comparison of couples accompanied and unaccompanied by children. *Journal of Marriage and the Family,* 1974, *36,* 750-755.

Rosenthal, R. *Experimenter effects in behavioral research.* New York: Appleton-Century-Crofts, 1966.

Roskies, E., & Lazarus, R. Coping theory and the teaching of coping skills. In P.O. Davidson & S.M. Davidson (Eds.), *Behavioral medicine: Changing health lifestyles.* New York: Brunner/Mazel, 1980.

Ross, L., & Sawhill, V. *Time of transition: The growth of families headed by women.* Washington, DC: The Urban Institute, 1975.

Rossi, A.S. A good woman is hard to find. *Trans-Action,* 1964, *2,* 20-23.

Rossi, A.S. Transition to parenthood. *Journal of Marriage and the Family*, 1968, *30*, 26-39.

Rotter, J. Generalized expectancies for internal versus external control of reinforcement. *Psychological Monographs*, 1966, 80.

Rowe, M. Choosing child care: Many options. In R. Rapoport & R. Rapoport (Eds.), *Working couples*. New York: Harper & Row, 1978.

Russell, C.S. Transition to parenthood: Problems and gratifications. *Journal of Marriage and the Family*, 1974, *36*, 294-302.

Ryder, R.G. Longitudinal data relating marriage satisfaction and having a child. *Journal of Marriage and the Family*, 1973, *35*, 604-607.

Sager, C.J. *Marriage contracts and couple therapy*. New York: Brunner/Mazel, 1976.

Sanguilano, I. *In her time*. New York: William Morrow and Company, 1978.

Satir, V. *Conjoint family therapy: A guide to theory and technique*. Palo Alto, CA: Science and Behavior Books, 1964.

Schumm, W.R., & Bollman, S.R. Interpersonal processes in rural families. In R.T. Coward & W.M. Smith, Jr. (Eds.), *The family in rural society*. Boulder, CO: Westview Press, 1981, 129-146.

Schwarzweller, H.K., & Crowe, J.M. Adaptation of Appalachian migrants to an industrial work situation: A case study. In E.B. Brody (Ed.), *Behavior in new environments: Adaptation of migrant populations*. Beverly Hills, CA: Sage Publications, 1969.

Seiden, A. Time management and the dual-career couple. In F. Pepitone-Rockwell (Ed.), *Dual-career couples*. Beverly Hills, CA: Sage Publications, 1980.

Seidenberg, R. *Corporate wives—corporate casualties*. New York: American Management Association, 1973.

Sell, K.D. *Joint custody and coparenting*. Paper presented at National Council on Family Relations, August 1979.

Selye, H. *The stress of life*. New York: McGraw-Hill, 1956.

Selye, H. *Stress without distress*. Philadelphia, PA: Lippincott & Crowell, 1974.

Selye, H. On the real benefits of eustress. *Psychology Today*, March 1978, *11*, 60.

Sheehy, G. *Passages: Predictable crises of adult life*. New York: Pantheon Books, 1976.

Simon, A. *Stepchild in the family: A view of children in remarriage*. New York: Odyssey Press, 1964.

Silverstone, B., & Hyman, H. *You and your aging parent*. New York: Pantheon Books, 1976.

Smith, R.M., & Smith, C.W. Child-rearing and single-parent fathers. *Family Relations*, 1981, *30*, 411-417.

Sollie, D.L., & Miller, B.C. The transition to parenthood as a critical time for building family strengths. In N. Stinnett, B. Chesser, H. DeFrain, & P. Knaub (Eds.), *Family strengths: Positive models for family life*. Lincoln, NE: University of Nebraska Press, 1980.

Solomon, E. *The anxious economy*. San Francisco: W.H. Freeman, 1975.

Spanier, G.B., & Casto, R.F. *Adjustment to separation and divorce: A qualitative analysis*. Unpublished manuscript. The Pennsylvania State University, 1977.

Speer, D.C. Family systems: Morphostasis or morphogenesis, or is homeostasis enough? *Family Process*, 1970, *9*, 259-278.

Sprenkle, D.H., & Olson, D.H. Circumplex model of marital and family systems IV: Empirical study of clinic and non-clinic couples. *Journal of Marital and Family Therapy*, 1978, *4*, 58-74.

Stack, C. *All our kin*. New York: Harper & Row, 1975.

Staples, R. *The Black family: Essays and studies*. Belmont, CA: Wadsworth Publishing Company, 1971.

Steffensmeier, R.H. *A role analysis of the transition to parenthood: Research continuities and further developments*. Doctoral dissertation. University of Iowa, 1977. Ann Arbor, MI: University Microfilms International, 1978.

Stein, P. *Single*. Englewood Cliffs, NJ: Prentice-Hall, 1976.

Stein, R.L. The economic statistics of families headed by women. *Monthly Labor Review*, January 1970, *93*, 3-8.

Stierlin, H. *Separating parents and adolescents.* New York: Quadrangle, 1974.

Stinnett, N. In search of strong families. In N. Stinnett, B. Chesser, & J. DeFrain (Eds.), *Building family strengths: Blueprints for action.* Lincoln, NE: University of Nebraska Press, 1979.

Sullivan, S. *The father's almanac.* New York: Doubleday & Company, 1980.

Sussman, M. The family life of older people. In R.H. Binstock & E. Shanas (Eds.), *Handbook on aging and the social sciences.* New York: Van Nostrand Reinhold, 1976.

Tenhouten, W. The Black family: Myth and reality. *Psychiatry,* May 1970, *2,* 145-173.

Tew, J., Laurence, K., Payne, H., & Rawnsley, K. Marital stability following the birth of a child with spina bifida. *British Journal of Psychiatry,* 1977, *131,* 79-82.

Toffler, A. *Future shock.* New York: Random House, 1970.

Tremblay, K.R., Jr., Walker, F.S., & Dillman, D.A. The quality of life experienced by rural families. In R.T. Coward & W.M. Smith, Jr. (Eds.), *Serving families in rural America: Program design and delivery.* Lincoln, NE: University of Nebraska Press, 1983.

Troll, L. The family of later life: A decade review. *Journal of Marriage and the Family,* 1971, *33,* 263-290.

Uhlmann, J.M. Boom towns: Implications for human services. In M.O. Wagenfeld (Ed.), *Perspectives on rural mental health.* San Francisco, CA: Jossey-Bass, 1981.

Unger, D.G., & Powell, D.R. Supporting families under stress: The role of social networks. *Family Relations,* 1980, *9,* 566-574.

United States Bureau of the Census. Social and economic characteristics of the metropolitan and nonmetropolitan population: 1977 and 1970. (*Current Population Reports,* P-25, No. 15). Washington, DC: U.S. Government Printing Office, 1978.

United States Bureau of the Census. Characteristics of the population below the poverty level: 1978. (*Current Population Reports,* Series P-60, No. 124). Washington, DC: U.S. Government Printing Office 1980.(a)

United States Bureau of the Census. Household and family characteristics: March 1979. (*Current Population Reports,* Series P-20, No. 352). Washington, DC: U.S. Government Printing Office, 1980.(b)

United States Bureau of the Census. Population profile of the United States: 1980. (*Current Population Reports,* Series P-20, No. 363). Washington, DC: U.S. Government Printing Office, 1980.(c)

United States Bureau of the Census. Characteristics of households and persons receiving noncash benefits: 1979. (*Current Population Reports,* Series P-23, No. 110). Washington, DC: U.S. Government Printing Office, 1981. (a)

United States Bureau of the Census. Money income and poverty status of families and persons in the United States, 1980. (*Current Population Reports,* Series P-60, No. 127). Washington, DC: U.S. Government Printing Office, 1981. (b)

United States Bureau of Labor Statistics. *The consumer price index: Concepts and content over the years.* Washington, DC: U.S. Government Printing Office, 1978.

United States Bureau of Labor Statistics. *CPI Issues.* Washington, DC: U.S. Government Printing Office, 1980. (a)

United States Bureau of Labor Statistics. *Handbook of labor statistics.* (Bulletin 2070). Washington, DC: U.S. Government Printing Office, 1980. (b)

United States Bureau of Labor Statistics. *Perspectives on working women: A databook.* Washington, DC: U.S. Government Printing Office, 1980. (c)

United States Department of Agriculture. *A time to choose: Summary report on the structure of agriculture.* (Publication Number 723-560-686). Washington, DC: U.S. Government Printing Office, 1981.

Ursin, H., Baade, E., & Levine, S. (Eds.) *Psychobiology of stress: A study of coping men.* New York: Academic Press, 1978.

Veevers, J.E., & Figley, C.R. *Childless by choice.* Toronto, Canada: Butterworths, 1980.

Verhulst, J., & Heiman, J. An interactional approach to sexual dysfunctions. *American Journal of Family Therapy,* 1979, *7,* 19-36.

Vincent, C.E. Familia spongia: The adaptive function. *Journal of Marriage and the Family,* 1966, *28,* 29-36.

Visher, E., & Visher, J. Common problems of stepparents and their spouses. *American Journal of Orthopsychiatry,* 1978, *48,* 252-262.

Visher, E., & Visher, J. *Stepfamilies: A guide to working with stepparents and stepchildren.* New York: Brunner/Mazel, 1979.

Vogel, E.F., & Bell, N.W. The emotionally disturbed child as the family scapegoat. In N. Bell & E. Vogel (Eds.), *A modern introduction to the family.* New York: The Free Press, 1968, 412-427.

Walker, K.M., MacBride, A., & Vachon, M.L.S. Social support networks and the crisis of bereavement. *Social Science and Medicine,* 1977, *11,* 35-41.

Walker, K., & Woods, M. *Time use: A measure of household production of family goods and services.* American Home Economics Association, 1976.

Waller, W. *The old love and the new.* Carbondale, IL: Southern Illinois University Press, 1958.

Wallerstein, J.S., & Kelly, J.B. The effects of parental divorce: The adolescent experience. In E.J. Anthony, & C. Koupernik (Eds.), *The child in his family: Children at psychiatric risk III.* New York: John Wiley & Sons, 1974.

Wallerstein, J.S., & Kelly, J.B. The effects of parental divorce: Experiences of the preschool child. *American Academy of Psychiatry,* 1975, *14,* 600-616.

Wallerstein, J.S., & Kelly, J.B. The effects of parental divorce: Experiences of the child in early latency. *American Journal of Orthopsychiatry,* 1976, *46,* 20-32.

Wallerstein, J.S., & Kelly, J.B. Divorce counseling: A community service for families in the midst of divorce. *American Journal of Orthopsychiatry,* 1977, *47,* 4-22.

Wallerstein, J.S., & Kelly, J.B. California's children of divorce. *Psychology Today,* 1980, *13,* 67-76.

Wandersman, L.P. Parenting groups to support the adjustment to parenthood. *Family Perspective,* 1978, *12,* 117-120.

Wandersman, L.P. The adjustment of fathers to their first baby. *Birth and the Family Journal,* 1980, *7,* 155-162.

Wandersman, L.P. *Supportive parent education programs: What are we learning?* Paper presented at the Society for Research in Child Development Biennial Meeting, Boston, Mass., April 1981.

Weinberg, J.S. Body image disturbance as a factor in the crisis situation of preganancy. *Journal of Obstetric and Gynecologic Nursing.* 1978, *7,* 18-21.

Weiss, R.S. *Marital separation.* New York: Basic Books, 1975.

Weiss, R.S. The emotional impact of marital separation. *Journal of Social Issues,* 1976, *32,* 135-146.

Weiss, R.S. *Going it Alone.* New York: The Free Press, 1980.

Wells, R.V. Demographic change and the life cycle of American families. In T.K. Rabb & R.I. Rotberg (Eds.), *The family in history.* New York: Harper & Row, 1973.

Westin, J. *Making do: How women survived in the 1930s.* Chicago, IL: Follet, 1976.

Westman, J. Effect of divorce on children's personality development. *Medical Aspects of Human Sexuality,* 1972, *6,* 38-55.

Westoff, L.A. *The second time around: Remarriage in America.* New York: Viking Press, 1977.

White, A. *Factors making for difficulties in the stepparent relationship with children* (Abstract of a thesis). Illinois Institute for Juvenile Research, 1943.

Whiteside, M., & Auerbach, L. Can the daughter of my father's new wife be my sister? Families of remarriage in family therapy. *Journal of Divorce,* 1978, *1,* 271-283.

Wilkening, E.A. Farm families and family farming. In R.T. Coward & W.M. Smith, Jr. (Eds.), *The family in rural society.* Boulder, CO: Westview Press, 1981.

Winch, R.F., & Greer, S. Urbanism, ethnicity and extended familism. *Journal of Marriage and the Family.* 1968, *30,* 40-45.

Wingspread Report. *Strengthening families through informal support systems.* Racine, WI: The

Johnson Foundation, 1978.

Wiseman, R. Crisis theory and the process of divorce. *Social Casework*, 1975, 56 (4), 205-212.

Woods, N.F. *Human sexuality in health and illness.* St. Louis, MO: The C.V. Mosby Company, 1979.

Working Family Project. Parenting. In R. Rapoport & R. Rapoport (Eds.), *Working couples.* New York: Harper & Row, 1978.

Yankelovich, D. *New rules: Searching for self-fulfillment in a world turned upside down.* New York: Random House, 1981.

Young, L. *Wednesday's children.* New York: McGraw-Hill Book Company, 1964.

Zawadski, B., & Lazarsfeld, P. The psychological consequences of unemployment. *Journal of Social Psychology*, 1935, 6, 224-251.

Zur-Szpiro, S., & Longfellow, C. *Support from fathers: Implications for the well-being of mothers and their children.* Paper presented at the Society for Research in Child Development Biennial Meeting, Boston, April 1981.

Name Index, Volumes I and II

247

Subject Index, Volumes I and II